The
Yoga
of
Food

About the Author

Melissa Grabau, PhD (Sacramento, CA), received her doctorate in Clinical Psychology from Duquesne University in 1998. She became licensed as a psychologist in California in 2001 and has been in private practice since 2003. More recently, she has broadened her existential/humanistic background in psychology to incorporate her long-standing interest in yoga and Eastern psychology. She is a certified yoga teacher and currently integrates mind-body techniques in her work with clients. For more information, visit witnesstherapy.com.

To Write the Author

If you wish to contact the author or would like more information about this book, please write to the author in care of Llewellyn Worldwide, and we will forward your request. Both the author and the publisher appreciate hearing from you and learning of your enjoyment of this book and how it has helped you. Llewellyn Worldwide cannot guarantee that every letter written to the author can be answered, but all will be forwarded. Please write to:

Melissa Grabau, PhD
℅ Llewellyn Worldwide
2143 Wooddale Drive
Woodbury, MN 55125-2989

Please enclose a self-addressed stamped envelope for reply,
or $1.00 to cover costs. If outside the USA, enclose
an international postal reply coupon.

Many of Llewellyn's authors have websites with additional information and resources. For more information, please visit www.llewellyn.com.

The Yoga of Food

Wellness from the Inside Out

Healing the
Relationship with
Food & Your
Body

Melissa Grabau, PhD

Llewellyn Publications
Woodbury, Minnesota

FIRST EDITION
Second Printing, 2014

Book design by Bob Gaul
Cover design by Lisa Novak
Cover illustration by Christiane Beauregard/Lindgren & Smith
Excerpts reprinted from: *LIGHT ON LIFE* by B.K.S. Iyengar. Copyright © 2005
  by B.K.S. Iyengar. Permission granted by Rodale, Inc., Emmaus, PA 18098.
Editing by Ed Day

Llewellyn Publications is a registered trademark of Llewellyn Worldwide Ltd.

Library of Congress Cataloging-in-Publication Data (Pending)
978-0-7387-4015-7

Llewellyn Worldwide Ltd. does not participate in, endorse, or have any authority or responsibility concerning private business transactions between our authors and the public.

All mail addressed to the author is forwarded, but the publisher cannot, unless specifically instructed by the author, give out an address or phone number.

Any Internet references contained in this work are current at publication time, but the publisher cannot guarantee that a specific location will continue to be maintained. Please refer to the publisher's website for links to authors' websites and other sources.

Llewellyn Publications
A Division of Llewellyn Worldwide Ltd.
2143 Wooddale Drive
Woodbury, MN 55125-2989
www.llewellyn.com

Printed in the United States of America

5617

Contents

Part Three: The Workings of Your Mind—Let's Dig In

Acknowledgements

I am deeply indebted to the individuals who allowed me to use their stories in this book. Without all of you, this book would not have been possible. Melissa Flashman, thank you for seeing potential in my manuscript and for your intelligent and positive direction. Angela Wix, your intuitive sense of what this book could be brought it to a new level. Thank you. Ed Day, such appreciation for your responsive collaboration and your attention to detail. Finally, thank you to Karen Miscall-Bannon for your careful reading and sharing your deep, accurate knowledge of yoga philosophy.

Dedication

Mark and Rachel. I love you both.

Introduction:
Yoga as a Guide for Living and Eating Well

Nine o'clock a.m. Amanda is late for therapy. I hear the overtones of exasperation in her voicemail. She recounts her frustration later on in the session. The planning she put into being on time. Her anger when traffic foiled her plans. The pervasiveness of anger in the rest of her life. This is concerning and bewildering to her since she says she has never felt anger before, even in the face of her mother's cruel and unpredictable rages.

Amanda is thirty years old, with two young children, a husband, financial problems, and a lot of anxiety. She arrives neatly dressed, with her long brown hair pulled back in a tight braid that nicely frames her round, pleasant face. She looks professional, put together, albeit carrying more weight than she would like for her 5-foot-4 frame. Her voice is resonant with feeling and her words are elegantly articulated as she recounts further frustration with plans that have gone awry. "My husband called yesterday and suggested that we go out to celebrate my birthday that night rather than Thursday. I thought, 'Why not? I'd been good all day.' And the day had gone really well. I'm feeling better at my job. Nobody yelled at me today, and that's a good day. We went to the Outback Steak House." She went on to describe the meal laden with carbohydrates and fat. "First they brought out a big plate of potato skins, then bread and salad with ranch dressing. Then the steak with fries. And then, because it was my birthday, they brought a cake!" She looks defeated as she expresses her bewilderment at her lack of resolve, the collapse of her good day and mood as she left the restaurant with her little girls and husband, and a body that felt heavy and bloated.

Let's pause here for a moment and sweep this very ordinary scene with an inquisitive eye. Perhaps you recognize yourself in both Amanda's good intentions and impending demoralization. Perhaps you often ask yourself why it is that despite your best intentions, you too repeatedly become derailed at the dinner table. By probing beneath the surface of this brief, seemingly inconsequential scene from Amanda's life, you just might come to understand how it is that amidst the immediate stressors and background dramas that populate our day-to-day lives, the dinner table can take on so much magnitude. It not only wields the power to warp precious moments of your life with indigestion and bloat, it can contribute to heart disease, diabetes, and premature death, which we all know may lurk ever so silently in the background.

In my work as a therapist, I hear stories. These stories are often stories about the body and chronicle the frustrations and anguish plaguing even the most privileged bodies on our planet. One of the themes that continually replays in my office is the heartache and demoralization felt by women and men of all ages and circumstances who struggle with their weight and their relationship to food. This is far more than a petty cosmetic problem. This is a problem that encapsulates one of our main challenges as modern human beings—learning how to live well in our bodies. This includes our ability to manage our hungers, to balance pleasure with restraint and good sense, and to regulate our energies so that we are able to face the challenges of daily life without collapse. How we feel day to day, our general health and energy levels, and our overall sense of safety and peace in our own flesh have an enormous impact on how we feel about ourselves and our capacity to function effectively in the world. So many of us, particularly women, are at war with our bodies. This internal rift pervades everything and compromises our sense of self and our presence with others. Our culture's obsession with dieting, combined with the health crisis obesity presents, is a pressing societal problem. It is most obviously a health issue. It is also a psychological issue due to the emotional suffering food and weight problems create. Fundamentally, it is a quality of life issue due to the enormous impact our nutritional habits have on our ability to live well.

The word *yoga* literally means "to yoke or unite." In yoga practice, we are often told that we are bringing together the mind with the breath or the body with the mind. The yoga of food means uniting the purpose of eating, nourishing the body and soul, with the practice and act of eating. Currently, there is a woeful discord between the actual purpose of eating—nourishment—and the act of eating, which for many of us can be negligent and, at times, even abusive toward the body. We may know in our heads that it is important to eat plenty of fruits and vegetables, high-quality protein, unsaturated fat, and so on, yet many of us continue to have a damnable time uniting this knowledge with actual changes in our eating habits. We are like Amanda, feeling pretty good and then sideswiped by a plate of food that leaves us speechless and uncomfortable in its wake. The good news is that you can approach this problem, which is both very personal, but also cultural, in a new way that will facilitate growth on many levels. You cannot and really should not do this work alone. We can extend the meaning of the word "yoga" to include an imperative to bring people and communities together to address the problem of our current nutritional habits and health status. We can and, I would argue, must unite in an effort to compassionately and tenaciously reconfigure our current culturally sanctioned self-care habits into saner and more sustainable nourishment for body, mind, and soul. Yoga provides a means to do this and this book will show you how, starting with you, the individual.

This book is less about the physical practice of yoga and more about its principles, introducing you to yoga philosophy with the intention of demonstrating how you can use this ancient discipline to facilitate changes in your patterns of eating and self-care. Yoga is uniquely designed to help you with these issues because its philosophical system, at least as it has evolved here in the West, is based on reverence for the physical body. In modern yogic philosophy, the body is envisaged as a reflection of universal intelligence. In order to become more responsive to this intelligence, you must practice shifting your awareness from the outside—measured by pounds and inches, to the inside, where an ocean of vitality and wisdom awaits your discovery.

This book is intended to be interactive, so I suggest that you purchase a journal and prepare yourself to be an active participant as you read. A lot of information here is intended for the beginning yoga student, and at the end of each chapter there are many opportunities for self-reflection. I am hoping that the information offered is accessible and understandable, even though much of it has esoteric origins. In spite of the esoteric nature of its roots, the ideas from yoga are astoundingly relevant to the human condition throughout the ages. It is my hope that the self-reflective exercises will help you to absorb and integrate the information so that it becomes knowledge, something that you know at the level of your experience, rather than merely interesting ideas that remain unrelated to your life.

The book is divided into three main sections. Part One describes your everyday sense of self that it is uninformed by a yogic perspective. Part Two introduces the yogic perspective on your body with the intention to help you relate to your physical, energetic, and mental bodies with a new appreciation. Part Three discusses the yogic perspective on your mind and shows how you can harness the power of your mind to enhance the change process. I pull heavily from B.K.S. Iyengar's book *Light on Life: The Yoga Journey to Wholeness, Inner Peace and Ultimate Freedom.* Following his lead, I use Sanskrit terminology throughout the text, but hopefully with enough explanation and context that the terms will not seem so foreign that you cannot relate them to your own experience. In all, this book is intended to be highly relatable to your life and a means to help you move beyond nonproductive and self-destructive habits, particularly as they manifest with food.

How I Came to Write This Book

I am the perfect person to write a book about the yoga of food. The reason has something to do with my education as a psychologist, but nothing to do with my "enviable" health or physique. The reason is not because I eat mindfully and gracefully—mind and body a synchronized symphony of reason melded with pleasure. No, sadly, more often than not I have been the gal sucking on a chicken bone while standing at the counter, ravenous and stressed, belching pitifully after having overeaten for the umpteenth time, carried away by hunger, greed, or just plain mindlessness. Throughout my life, I have followed many of the "rules" of good nutrition, however, the tide of untamed impulse and emotion beneath the rules will quickly hijack a life of good intentions and create enormous pain and dis-ease. I've lived it firsthand and seen it in those that I love.

Having benefited enormously from both the physical practice and the philosophical perspective of yoga, I am firmly entrenched on the healing path of yoga. I know that it is a practice that can help others who share similar difficulties living in their bodies and navigating our current culinary landscape. I originally aimed this book toward people with eating disorders, however, I have reconfigured the book toward a more general audience who, like me, are suffering from the seemingly benign guidelines of the Standard American Diet (SAD). I have come to believe that this way of eating is engineered to create sadness on many levels, mind, body, and soul. When coupled with a frantic lifestyle and a fixation upon the girth of the body, or numbers on the scale, it is a recipe for disaster. It is only when we stop seeing this way of eating and living as normal and desirable, believing that something is wrong with us because we just can't get it right, that we will begin to experience some freedom in our minds and bodies.

Yoga philosophy is geared toward freeing ourselves from our personal conditioning, as well as from the shared pitfalls of the human condition. There has been a blanket assumption in our culture that yoga practice, the poses, are inextricably linked to yoga philosophy. Recently, there has been a dawning awareness that that is just plain not true. Yoga philosophy, which is a technology of mind, is indeed thousands of years old. The physical practice that we know today is a modern invention from India, created in the early twentieth century. In her book *Yoga Ph.D.*, Carol Horton argues that this fact makes yoga no less meaningful or relevant for our current individual and collective needs. Rather, she asserts that it is the flexibility of yoga to morph and reshape itself to conform to the current demands and exigencies of our cultural milieu that gives yoga so much power. So while yoga philosophy and the physical practice are highly compatible, they do not necessarily need to come as a package deal. In this book, I do pull them together and attempt to show how they can create a synergistic power in your healing process.

My profession as a psychologist has been extremely helpful and pertinent in my endeavor to write this book. First of all, I am deeply beholden to the clients who have shared their personal stories with me. It is an honor to be entrusted with such raw, at times enormously painful, disclosures. I have been in the field of psychology, either learning or practicing, for over twenty-five years. Throughout these years, I have observed some consistent themes in human suffering, as well as in the change process. First of all, the realities of our current condition feel permanent. As much as we may know in our heads that change is possible, probable, indeed inevitable, it takes tremendous faith and courage to unhook from our current reality and engage in an intentional change process. Every time I receive a new client phone call, I know that it is someone who has reached a limit of suffering and, heart in throat, has picked up the phone and reached out. It is a precious moment charged with both pain and hope. And throughout the change process, hope and despair do a little dance. Enter hope, providing a light of possibility, a new perspective, a way to realign things so that we may be relieved of suffering. Then, unannounced and unsolicited, the siren call of old habits and former pleasures sounds and we are led off the path of change. We regress. We despair. We suffer. Then we remember the light of possibility briefly glimpsed and emboldened; we tentatively continue on the path of change. Back and forth, up and down, losing our way and staying the course. Over time, the regressions are less severe and predictable and faith in the process begins to take a stronger hold. Many of us fall off the path, however, and it is often a long time before the weight of suffering creates enough pressure to reengage with hope. This is always a good thing, but the longer we wait and the longer we engage in old habits, the more damages have accrued and the longer it takes to dig out. Meaning, we have to have ever more faith to stay the course the second, third, or fourth time around. I am hoping that outlining this dialectic around the process of changing eating and self-care habits will help feed your faith and courage as you navigate your own personal dialectic of hope and despair.

Along with being a psychologist, I have been a yoga practitioner and student for the past eleven years. In 2008, I attended a ten-month teacher training in Integrative Yoga Therapy. I was granted the luxury of spending a weekend a month in the charming town of Petaluma, California, where I was steeped in yoga theory and practice with a group of like-minded people. I have always been drawn to the wisdom of Eastern philosophy and my yoga training solidified my sense that Eastern traditions have a great deal to offer us in the West. As a psychotherapist, my emphasis has been on the psyche and the curative power of bringing language and stories to experience. And yet, behind all the stories is the unarticulated, and often unarticulatable (yes, I know that is not a word, though perhaps that underlines my point) realm of the body. Here, in this private world we all inhabit, we are subjected to alternating discomfort and satisfaction, pleasures and pains both large and small. These oscillations are governed by the rhythms of ongoing contraction and release that regulate all plant and animal life on the planet. Yoga theory is an affirmation of this hidden domain of the body and its interwoven layers of matter, energy, and thought. The yoga of food embraces the likeness our bodies share with the matter and energy of food and helps us utilize food's matter and energy to better nourish our bodies. According to yoga theory, we are more alike than different. And we have more in common with ladybugs, elephants, and apples, let alone with each other, than we might care to admit. This can actually be good news as we avail ourselves of an intelligence that is greater than our own and join with others with whom we are more alike than different. And perhaps this is the greatest takeaway that modern yoga has to offer us—we are not alone. We are connected to one another, the earth, and the stars, and we can take comfort and find guidance in this presence. And here is where yoga practice comes in—a pose is just a pose, but when the position of the body is guided by the focus of the mind, the inspiration of the breath, and the shared language of the sequences, it elevates to a beautiful medium through which to experience and explore our shared human Being. The connection generated by participating in this shared practice that is sweeping through our towns and suburbs affirms our shared humanity and can fuel our efforts to rise above our personal suffering and join a movement toward greater individual, and eventually global, health. The yoga of food seeks to bring this celebration of life beyond the mat to the dinner table in the humble process of together relearning to feed ourselves well.

Part One

Your Current Self-Understanding

The Foundation of Yoga, Food, and You

This first section encompasses chapter 1 and chapter 2. We will explore some basic concepts of yoga philosophy and introduce you to a yogic perspective on the human condition. We will touch on how these issues are relevant to your relationship to food; however, the meat of this section will focus on helping you understand and relate concepts from yoga philosophy to your own life and body.

Chapter One

Obstacles to "Clear Seeing" (The Kleshas)

Have you ever looked up on a clear night and upon seeing the star-spangled sky above felt a deep serenity and peace? Maybe you have looked into your child's eyes and sensed both your legacy and your continuity. Or you've had a friend diagnosed with an illness that made you suddenly and painfully aware of the fragility of life. I know you have had these experiences in some shape or form because I have had them too. This points to one of the main yogic principles—we are more alike than different. We are like snowflakes, each of us sharing an inherent structure that differs only in its finer points of articulation.

The experience of "clear seeing," a concept from yoga philosophy, are those moments when we are in touch with the magnitude of the universe and our small but precious place in it. The capacity for clear seeing is a uniquely human trait that we all experience from time to time throughout our lives.

Unfortunately, most of the time we tend to be so caught up in triviality and immediacy that we are not in touch with this larger perspective. We overlook what is truly important in life (our relationships, our health, spiritual meaning) and fall into the trap of seeking comfort, aggrandizement, and distraction through obtaining a new this or a new that, ever trying to appease our constantly shifting attention. When we are caught up in this way, we tend to make poor choices that create suffering. This tendency is not a problem unique to the twentieth or twenty-first centuries. B.K.S. Iyengar, one of India's famous yogis who is credited with bringing yoga to the United States, puts it this way in his book *Light on Life*: "Yoga recognizes that the way our bodies and minds work has changed very little over the millennia … there are inherent stresses, like geological fault lines that, left unaddressed, will always cause things to go wrong, whether individually or collectively."

The "inherent stressors" to which Iyengar refers are called the kleshas, which means "obstructions to clear seeing." Similar to our digestive systems, our basic psychic systems have changed little over time. Although the circumstances of our lives have changed drastically, the structure of human suffering has basically stayed the same. The kleshas, which underlie our tendency to go astray, are extraordinarily relevant to our modern struggle with food and health issues. So, although having an abundance of food and being overfed may be relatively new in the course of human evolution, the human frailties driving this problem are as old as the stars. By placing your individual food/body issues within this larger context, you refocus your attention from the details of your individual struggle, be it a fixation upon reaching a certain body size or an obsession with Oreo cookies, and instead you come to appreciate how your individual issues replay dramas experienced by humans throughout time.

Five Obstacles to "Clear Seeing"

1. Unclear Seeing

This is the root of all suffering. We are disconnected from the mystery and unity of the Universe, of which we are all a part. We take nature, our body, our life on this planet under the stars within the infinite, for granted. We are too busy counting pennies or calories, pinching extra flesh on our thighs, avoiding mirrors, and pleasing others. We are lost in our own ways of marking time, getting through the day and making it to a magical place in the future when we will finally be "happy." We don't notice what already is. We don't see.

2. Ego

Ego springs from the ground of unclear seeing. We feel ourselves as separate and disconnected from others and from the world. This leads to an overvaluation of Self. The world revolves around us. Our unhappiness, our struggles, our goals, our successes, feel large and all-important. We may be obsessed with our failures or obsessed with our imagined greatness. Either way, we discount others due to our self-absorption. We are preoccupied with "What's in it for me?" Pursuing and securing our own comforts and pleasure consumes us.

3. Attraction

We are drawn toward what feels good, or has made us feel good in the past. We attempt to pull things into our world that we associate with comfort, security, and good feelings. We seek out things that secure our identity and status. Some of us become obsessed with money, some with success, some with love, some with food, some with drugs and alcohol. No matter what our attraction du jour may be, life becomes imbued with the need to control circumstances so that we are comfortable and pleasured. Why does this not lead to happiness?

4. Aversion

We recoil from things we associate with pain or believe threatens our identity. Our lives become structured around avoiding what is unpleasant and garnering what is pleasant. What is wrong with this? Nothing, except that it doesn't work. Life is uncertain. When we attempt to control circumstances so that we remain comfortable, we are engaged in an unwinnable project. This is why so many of us become "control freaks." We are "freaks" because we are going against an organizing principle of the universe—life is uncertain and we are not meant to be perpetually comfortable. The more we insist on always feeling good, the more miserable we become.

5. Fear

We live in fear. Fear of loss, and ultimately fear of death. Fear of recognition of our transience on the earth. Our presence on the earth is very fleeting and our all-important Self is really not all that important. So we pursue pleasure and avoid pain and get through the day. We avoid recognition of our vulnerability and lose ourselves in the illusion of the everyday.

Showing the Kleshas in Action

Unclear seeing is the mother of all the kleshas. It refers to the deeply human tendency to lose perspective about what is truly important and gives birth to our attachments, our self-preoccupation, and our fears. When we get lost in a small perspective, it is very easy to forget our blessings, our values, and the impact of our choices. When I go to a yoga class, the teacher will often begin by suggesting that we set an intention for our practice. This suggestion recalls us to ourselves and reminds us of our capacity to direct our conscious thoughts and behavior toward an intended outcome. We cannot control our thoughts or feelings, but we can coax our minds and bodies toward certain tendencies and ideas. We can actively choose what we wish to cultivate in our practice and in our lives. The practice of setting an intention acts as an antidote to unclear seeing.

Unclear seeing, as it relates to food and our bodies, is getting so lost in the "shoulds" and "shouldn'ts," followed by self-reproach and criticism, that we aren't even aware we are lost. Then we reinforce the negativity by skipping yoga and ignoring, denying, and avoiding the realities of our flesh with unhealthy, numbing behaviors (overeating and overdrinking are common examples). Our unclear seeing is perpetuated in our schizophrenigenic food culture, where we are teased and tempted by sumptuous, tantalizing foods, coupled with images of impossibly sculpted and honed bodies, all the while being inundated with health information informing us of the dire consequences of our current culturally sanctioned habits. This leads to a negative, fear-based relationship with our bodies. "What's wrong with me that I just ate that cookie?" This sentiment is just the tip of the iceberg of negativity that abounds regarding our flesh. On the flip side are the people who obsessively restrict food and drive their exhausted bodies through punishing exercise regimens, seeking an ideal that rests on a daily grind that verges on tortuous. Neither tactic is a good way to live, and both reflect a culture that is deeply confused.

The yoga of food will help you interrupt this pattern of negativity by showing you how to consciously introduce a more loving and accepting attitude toward your body. Just today I heard a yoga teacher tell the class that they had already done the hardest part—showing up. And that is the truth. Getting to your yoga class, breathing, and setting an intention to cut through the criticism with even just one small affirmation provides an opening to begin relating to your body as an expression of divine intelligence that deserves care, as opposed to a disappointing object of your judgment.

Unclear seeing is common to all human experience; however, when an individual has experienced relational trauma or abandonment, the tendency sets in earlier and more tenaciously. Dysfunctional attachment, also known as attraction and aversion, takes a stronger hold due to emotional/relational pain and misguided attempts to soothe that pain. When the world fails to be a secure and predictable place, attachments, ego, and fear gain more traction in the psyche. We attach to things to help cope with circumstances beyond our control and feelings that we are unable to handle or give voice to on our own.

When I was a young girl, about twelve years old, food became my life preserver. This was not something I consciously chose; it was as natural as drinking water when thirsty. I had a very close, symbiotic relationship with my mother. I was a shy, anxious child and she was my security. And then she left. Just for a month. A month for a twelve-year-old is long indeed. My father, struggling with major depression and his disintegrating marriage, withdrew into the comfort Walter Cronkite and a few drinks provided. My brother? Angry and confused, he got into something like four car accidents that year. And me? I went to school, where I felt relegated to the smart but unattractive group, came home and kerplunked in front of the TV. There I found comfort—*Gilligan's Island, The Brady Bunch, I Dream of Jeannie*... I had a crush on Bobby, wanted to be like Ginger, then Marsha, loved Jan's long blond hair, and coveted Jeannie's elegant yet cozy bedroom. Oh yes... and I ate. This was the '70s, which was a blessing because there were far fewer junk food options than there are today. Mozzarella cheese with saltine crackers (lots of them), a big bowl of Rice Krispies or Corn Flakes (with sugar), Dannon yogurt (fruit on the bottom), salami sandwiches on buttered, toasted bread... I once ate a whole frozen pizza for dinner during just one TV show. But at the time, there was no guilt. I was not yet particularly overweight and hadn't yet associated food with misery. It was comfort, which I turned to, an old friend to keep me company and soothe a sorrow that I could not even articulate. When I ate the pizza, I remember being surprised but not ashamed. It was a novelty at the time, yet it felt natural.

Understanding this through the lens of yoga, it is clear that I naturally turned toward something that had given me comfort in the past. Why do some of us choose food while others choose alcohol, or cigarettes, or sex? These are the particular articulations of the snowflake. The turning toward, however, is deeply human. We are attracted to what we associate with comfort. And as my experience so clearly illustrates, this is not a conscious choice. It is like drinking water when thirsty.

Food is a lovely feature of life on this planet. It feels really good to eat when hungry. I remember being a young girl, before life became stark and unfriendly, playing vigorously out in the expanse of meadow and trees in rural Vermont. I would make a pit stop at the house, red-cheeked and alive, a cool glass of milk gulped down with warm toast and melted peanut butter. And I was off again to play in the fields without a lingering thought given to my snack. Then there was the smell of my mother's fried chicken when our home felt safe and warm, the starry night outside, the anticipation of a delicious dinner inside. And these are only the conscious memories. Think of the infant, made irritable and uncomfortable from the nameless emptiness inside, who is then picked up and held, swallowing down warm, soothing milk. For some of us, many of us, food is intimately associated with warmth, comfort, and safety. And we turn to it as naturally as one who is thirsty turns to water.

Attraction and aversion are simple concepts, and yet, in my experience as a psychologist and a person, they explain much of what we see when we examine human behavior. We all want to feel good. We abhor feeling bad. And so we seek out whatever makes us feel good. If our ability to see clearly, which is already problematic given the fact that we are human, is further clouded by trauma, rejection, and other forms of emotional pain, we will fixate on inanimate things and on ourselves in order to cope with an unpredictable, difficult world. If we are unable to get our basic needs for acceptance and confidence met, we are vulnerable to fixating on something to substitute. If we feel strange and awkward with our peers, excluded from the joys of finding pleasure and competence in our work or play, we can turn to the act of chewing and swallowing to bind the fragments of our experience. In my description of eating the peanut butter toast, this was a natural, pleasurable activity that was secondary to the joy of playing outside. In contrast, eating in front of the TV was the experience in and of itself. The magnetic pull of attraction ("I want to feel good") became hooked to the feeling of comfort derived from chewing and swallowing due to the lack of other, more developmentally appropriate pleasures.

Now enter ego. Ego can be used both pejoratively (as in, "He has such a big ego"), while also describing a basic function of the mind. For Freud, ego is the mediator between the id, instinctual needs, and the superego, or conscience. In short, the ego introduces the reality principle—your ability to meet your needs (id) in a way that is respectful of societal prohibitions (superego). You must have an ego in order to function effectively in the world. Otherwise, you are at the mercy of your id ("I want it and I want it now!"), while simultaneously being battered by your superego ("You bad, bad girl, you should be ashamed!"). Think about it this way—your ego gets you out of bed in the morning when you would rather sleep in. Your ego gets you to balance your checkbook and do your taxes. You might imagine the dialogue (or "trialogue") like this: Id says, "Oh, this bed feels so good and warm. I want to lie here all day." Superego (of a punitive nature, not all superegos are punitive) chimes in, "Okay now, you lazy @#$%$. Get out of bed now and face up to your responsibilities! What were you thinking staying up so late?" Hopefully ego steps in now to mediate: "Okay, it's time to get up. You certainly are tired today, but you'll feel better once you start moving. Maybe you should think about going to bed a little earlier." But when the voices of the id and superego are too loud, the ego's voice can get lost. When you have a well-functioning ego, its voice is louder than the others and consequently, you experience less psychological conflict. Your id is less ravenous and insistent because she is confident her needs will be met ("All in good time, my dear") and your superego is able to lighten up a bit because she is confident that her expectations for order and civility will be respected.

In contrast to this psychological view of ego, in Classical Yoga philosophy, ego is something to be dissolved through the assiduous practice of meditation. Ego is envisaged as an ever-hungry, insatiable aspect of the self which convinces you that you are separate from others and perpetuates unclear seeing and suffering. It is desirable to be "ego-less" and the practices aim to quell the ego's incessant desires. Tantric Yoga philosophy is an out-growth of Classical Yoga and is more accepting of the body and the ego. Ego is not deemed something bad to "get rid of," but rather as a necessary part of your Being which you can harness toward action that is truly beneficial to you. In my opinion, this is a vital aspect of having a healthy self. Most of us can't, and speaking for myself, don't want to become ego-less. The question is: Is your ego in the service of trying to be "special," "better than," "thinner than … "? Or is your ego working to help you become a stronger, more vital, and loving person? If the former is your primary motivation, it is not "bad." However, being "better than," or striving to prove something to yourself or others is not a sustainable motivator and will eventually lead to further alienation from yourself and your flesh.

Let's explore how the misguided ego can get caught up in a food/body is-sues in a self-perpetuating, negative way. For most people, especially women, self-esteem is severely challenged by feeling overweight and being out of con-trol around food. It is easy to fixate on the fantasy that by losing weight and "controlling" yourself, you will fix all of your problems and restore your self-esteem. You focus your precious energies on perfecting your body in order to, well, perfect your body because you are under the delusion that this will perfect your self. This creates a futile preoccupation that is disconnected from any real love or appreciation for yourself, instead being in the service of a fantasy of control and attachment to an unrealistic image of yourself.

I vividly remember the pain of being caught in the cyclical delusion that obtaining body perfection was possible and would relieve me of the weight of being myself. When I was larger bodied in adolescence, a time of extreme self-consciousness for everyone, I felt very ashamed of my body, inferior to other girls, and defective around boys. Body competence is one of the main ways young people measure themselves against others, and when you are larger bodied, it can feel like a major strike against you. Some girls have enough intelligence and charisma to make up for this, but that certainly was not me. Feeling defective physically perpetuated my wavering sense of self-worth and competence. My ego was unable to effectively mediate my needs/impulses ("I want/need comfort!") and the demands of the external world ("Be socially and physically competent!"). This precipitated withdrawal from the world of my peers into a world of fantasy—"When I am thin…" Images of myself in tight jeans, high heels, and long hair populated my inner world. Redemption was just a few months of starvation away. My awkwardness and insecurity would all be fixed as I floated along in my new thin, ethereal body. One cannot live on fantasy alone, so in the real world I comforted myself with food. I soothed myself with the only comfort I knew, which sadly, only reinforced my conviction of defectiveness. This is the trap that many food overvaluators find themselves in—unable to get what you need in the world, you turn to food in order to find solace, which leaves you more depleted and dependent upon food to meet your needs. The same pattern holds for all addictive behaviors, including food-restrictors, who are caught in a self-reinforcing battle for control which it looks like they are "winning." This is very dangerous indeed because "winning" the battle for control by being thin masks the underlying desperation of the addiction. The fantasy, whether it be of "someday when I am thin," or of ultimate mastery of the body, perpetuates increasing isolation and self-focus. The fixation on yourself is fueled by your inability to function effectively in the world, creating quite a bit of egotism, though in the sense of self-absorption rather than grandiosity.

At the first stage, yoga is designed to build ego strength by enhancing your ability to connect with, rather than dissociate from, the realities of your body. You learn to face the substance of your body in the here and now and to open up windows and doorways through your own effort as you create new possibilities in your flesh. It can feel good at times and it can also be painful and demoralizing. This dialectic is like anything in life and it is essential to any change process. You toggle back and forth between your efforts and the inherent rewards in facing challenges in your life and your setbacks with their bitter disappointments. The point is that as you stay with the process, sometimes by virtue of blind faith, you build commitment to the practice, and over time the practice begins to seep into your bones. The term "ego strength" refers to your capacity to contend with reality and not retreat into your world of fantasy. Iyengar tells us that he has been known to slap a man's thigh and exclaim—"Willpower is here!" Ego strength, like willpower, is embodied. It builds over time through action. What better canvas than your own body to develop these qualities of willpower and ego strength?

The caveat here is for women who go too far on the other side of "using" the body as a canvas to display ego-strength and self-control. This applies to women who tend to overexercise, who are anorexic or "orthorexic" (a term for people obsessed with healthy eating). One can go too far into pushing and perfecting the body and thereby perpetuate a different kind of pain based on an unrealistic wish to overcome the body and its incessant needs and desires. The ego becomes an ever stronger, more rigid proponent of dominating the body. Again, yoga, when practiced in the spirit of yoga, is designed to honor and accommodate, as well as to challenge and expand the limits of the body. Nowadays, when I am in a class with some teachers, I notice that they are often the ones who will drop into child's pose and rest during a practice. Misguided, "willful" ego demands, "More!" "Harder!" "Faster!" Learning to listen to and allow a dialogue between ego and flesh is vital to the healing process. When ego is in the service of healing, it might mean pushing harder, or it might mean backing off. I wish I could give you a flow chart to let you know which to do when. Usually it's the less comfortable, less familiar course of action. As you get more accustomed to looking inside and listening to your flesh rather than your ego, you will gradually trust yourself to know what to do and when. You become more flexible, mind and body working together.

The final klesha is fear. Most broadly, this is conceptualized as fear of death. On a more day-to-day level, it is fear of loss of control. Many of my clients with food/body issues live with a strong buzz of fear just beneath the surface. Fear of illness, abandonment, helplessness, and financial destitution hover around the edges of the food. For them, the uncertainly of life in this body, on this planet, is intolerable. The fixation on food then becomes both the comfort in the midst of fear as well as the uncontrollable thing that eventually, tomorrow, next week, next diet, will be surmounted. Or, for the food restrictor, the daily "victories" with food and their body reinforces the misguided illusion of control. Both sides promise respite from the fear. In the meantime, a false sense of control is gained through the food—after all, you are the one who is doing this to yourself. You are not at the mercy of the universe but rather at the mercy of your own dysfunction.

For me, letting go of fear began (it is a process, not a switch that is flipped) when I stopped dieting and bingeing. Stopping dieting was even harder than stopping bingeing because it required letting go of the fantasy of quick and effortless redemption. This required me to begin facing my awkwardness with my peers, my discomfort in my body, and my raging insecurity without the buffer of my fantasy life and my food life. The kind of letting go I am describing here is a far cry from letting go of life and facing the fears most of us have of death. However, I think the two are related with regard to process, if not content. The process has to do with accepting inevitabilities of living life in the world, in a body constrained by basic laws of nature. At the level I am currently discussing, I had to accept that the body and life of my fantasy was just that—fantasy. I had to begin living in the world. This was not easy. And it was not a one, two, done process where you see awkward, overweight, and self-absorbed girl transformed into someone new, charming and likable in the next frame. It took many years of subsequent therapy, graduate school, and failed relationships—and the process is still not done. At every level of development, there are new challenges that require further peeling away, further letting go.

As you enter and progress through this book, you can expect to meet many different expressions of your self. You will confront your fears and regrets, and you will find your strength and compassion. Letting go of the past (who you have known yourself to be) and letting go of your current comforts is not easy. Nonetheless, there is a "rightness" to the process that you can use to guide and comfort yourself. By "rightness," I am referring to an implicit sense of direction and goodness that you will also taste frequently during this process. There is something that feels "right" about learning to live "life on life's terms." Another term for this is "alignment." When you are aligned with reality, more accepting of its constraints and possibilities, you just plain feel better.

Reflections on the Kleshas
Unclear Seeing

1. How often do you get in touch with a broader perspective regarding what really matters to you in life? An example might be when you talk to someone who inspires you and you think, "Yeah, that's how I would like to live." You are more in touch with your values at these times and feel willing to do the work to manifest these values in your life.

2. What circumstances or behaviors spark these experiences? Examples might be nature, death, cultural events, or reconnecting with old friends.

3. Does this sense of clarity change how you do things in your day-to-day life? In what way? How long does this change last?

4. What experiences or behaviors contribute to your unclear seeing? Alcohol use, overeating, violent movies, and being around certain people are possible examples.

Ego

1. How would you assess your ego strength on a scale of 1 to 5, with 5 being very strong? You can assess this with regard to your capacity to deal with reality in a straightforward way without retreating into fantasy or dramatizing small things. ("Oh my god, I gained 2 pounds!")

2. How strong is your sense of identity/self? Do you feel that you "know who you are"? Do you have clear values? Are you committed to various endeavors that give meaning to your life?

3. Do you feel that you are overly self-focused? Are there negative consequences to your self-absorption?

4. What commitments do you have that reach beyond your own comfort/security?

Attraction and Aversion

1. How do you please/comfort yourself on a daily basis? What gives you a feeling of security? Is there an unwelcome backlash to your comforts/security?

2. Do you have an addictive object/behavior? If so, when did this take root? What relational circumstances were you responding to when your fixation developed?

3. What do you try to avoid in your daily life? What techniques do you use to avoid? Examples are rationalization ("I deserve it, I've had a hard day"), procrastination ("I'll take care of it tomorrow"), or helplessness ("I just don't have the willpower").

4. How much difficulty does avoidance bring to your life? Examples might be stress related to a messy house, missed deadlines, or social isolation.

Fear

1. What are your biggest fears in life? How much do these fears curtail your day-to-day activities?

2. Are you a control freak? What do you try to control and how? What are the negative consequences of your efforts? Rigid

eating habits are a common example of over-control. Dislike of travel or fear of flying are other indicators of control issues.

3. How do you buffer yourself from your fears? Examples are avoidance of new activities, isolation, or overuse of alcohol or food.

4. Do you buffer against fear too much? How does your buffer get in the way of living more fully?

Your answers to these questions provide the backdrop for your ongoing inquiry as you proceed through the book. It is important to remind yourself of why you are seeking to heal your relationship with food and your body. From the perspective of yoga, this means living in harmony with the flow of life and freeing your energy so that you can participate more fully in this flow. The obstacles to clear seeing are obstacles to your flow. Healing your relationship with food is about your body, but it is ultimately to free you from bondage to your body so that you can become more involved in the process of life.

Chapter Two

Your Repeated Actions (Samskaras)

I have a bad habit of running late. I am a very early riser, but it seems that no matter how much time I have, I am always trying to beat the clock. It is both intentional and unintentional. "You're doing it again, Melissa," I chide myself as I insist on putting on lotion when I have to be out of the house in five minutes. "Why do you always do this to yourself?" I wonder as I thrust myself and my bags into my car and struggle to drive the speed limit, hoping that my first client may be running a bit late too. I cannot say that I have ever seriously tried to change this habit. It suits me somehow. My lifestyle has adjusted to this pattern and the habit reinforces these accommodations. Fitting that essential one last thing in is has become "just who I am," thank you very much.

Yoga theory has a term for power of habit in shaping who we are—*samskaras*. Samskaras are grooves in the body-mind that are created over time through repeated actions. This concept, psychologically speaking, reshapes and deepens our understanding of our habits from being merely pesky behavioral patterns that we should have the willpower to change, to a powerful force that has impact on us at material, energetic, and even a spiritual level. In other words, samskaras shed light on the apparent insanity of individuals who repeat self-destructive behavior over and over again, sometimes to the point of bringing about their own demise.

You Are What You Repeatedly Do

Samskaras create material and energetic conditions that strongly influence your current and future patterns of thoughts and behavior. On a material level, let's think about this in relation to the brain. You may have heard the phrase "Neurons that fire together wire together." Essentially, this means that through your repeated thoughts and behaviors, you create interstates in your brain—pathways that are paved and easily traveled due to your repeated use of them. You pave these highways, so to speak, by the repetition of certain thoughts and behaviors. The physical aspect of these highways is seen in your brain's increased myelination and neuronal growth in highly traveled pathways. A positive example of this is a musician who by virtue of repeated practice can allow the music to just flow through her effortlessly. With regard to eating habits, if you were raised in a home where you learned to eat reasonable portions of healthful food, this tendency will be so natural to you that it will be fairly easy for you to maintain this pattern for life. You may get derailed now and then, like gaining the "freshman 15" when you first leave home, but you will likely be able to interrupt the momentum of these bad habits relatively quickly. If, however, you have eaten larger and larger quantities of food over time and grown into a habit of binge eating, this pattern will be recorded in the wiring of your brain and the accommodations your body has made in response to this behavior. In both cases, your past behavior is written in your body and will have an influence on your present and future choices. The energetic field of these patterns, though less tangible, is equally, if not more important, than the material representation. The energetic field has to do with the thoughts and feelings, of which you are often not even aware, that drive and reinforce your behavioral pattern. Inarticulate longings for comfort, the strain of internal tension, and the unbearable weight of shame, fall into the less tangible, energetic field surrounding binge eating.

There are many useful metaphors for understanding samskaras. Sowing seeds in a garden is commonly used. Another metaphor is the image of a vehicle in a field driving in a circular path over and over and over again. The tire tracks would get pretty deep, making each subsequent lap easier. However, a different vehicle coming along with the intention of creating a new track would be hard-pressed to do so—breaking out of the ruts to create a new path on new terrain would take a lot of energy and intention. And this new path would feel unnatural and take a lot more energy to stay on. This is why habit change is so difficult. The grooves in your body and in your consciousness are deep. Staying within these grooves is comfortable, even when you know that the habits are detrimental to your health and well-being. In Iyengar's words: "In the end, we may accept the situation and just say, 'It's the way I am,' 'Life always lets me down,' 'Things just make me so angry,' or, 'I have an addictive personality.'" I phrase it this way: "We collapse into a heap of relief comingled with resigned despair. Maybe next time…" The problem is, with every collapse, "next time" is all the harder because you have just added to the groove of resignation.

Showing the Samskaras in Action

When I was caught in the samskara of a diet-binge cycle, I remember being desperate to stop my pattern of binge eating. This would be most acute after a binge, when I was suffused in a wake of hopelessness and shame wrought from my behavior. Periodically, I would muster up the resolve to go on a diet, determined this time not to "blow it" by giving in to the urge to binge. I would usually make it two or three days on a calorie-restricted diet. Then doubts in the form of vague whispers that had no words would start to edge in around my consciousness. I would push these whispers away, determined to be strong. Then something would happen. Either the press of hunger would become too much or I would experience something painful in my life that would push me over the edge. My drive to binge would be so strong and intense that I literally felt that I could not stop it. Even at the time, when I desperately wanted to be able to withstand the pull of the habit/samskara, I just could not do it. Relief and despair comingled in my frenzied awareness when I finally gave myself over to the sweetness of consumption.

Fast-forward a few years. I had gone through a lot of growth, having broken the symbiotic tie with my mother by spending a year at boarding school ("I can survive without her!"). I had stopped dieting for an extended period, which allowed me to regain some degree of normalcy in my eating habits. In addition, I had received some psychotherapy and gone on antidepressants. After all this, I had managed to lose about thirty-five pounds and now I was determined to keep it off. I was also determined not to stay on medication, as it threatened to put me in too close proximity to my father, who struggled with significant depression. I had slowly weaned from the medication and was on Thanksgiving break from boarding school, visiting my father in his condo, a community that was largely inhabited by college students. My father's unit was furnished with furniture from our past life in a country farmhouse, remnants of another world now lost to me. All the symbols of loss stored in this little condo were not in my conscious awareness. Food, however, all that it promised and all that was forbidden, was very present for me. We had gone for Thanksgiving dinner at some woman's house, one of my father's many "girlfriends" since the divorce. Her name was Carol. After dinner, my father and Carol went for a walk and I was left alone. I had exerted moderate control during the meal and was both sated and guilty, after all, it was more than usual. I felt drawn toward the refrigerator. I wanted to go and didn't want to go. There was a promise in there. Something exciting. It was chocolate crème pie that drew me. It is hard to describe both the lust and the pain that marks these moments of self-destruction. After all I had done, after not bingeing for over six months, after losing thirty-five pounds, the feeling was so strong that it felt like it was a force from outside of me. I was compelled. I got so far as digging the spoon into the cool creaminess of the pie, thrusting the spoon into my mouth, the energy of the binge was pulling me in with a strong, magnetic force. "NO!" An internal thrust gathered and broke through my mind into my body. "No!" I wrenched myself away from the refrigerator and outside into the air. I was full of pain, but also full of victory, because I knew that I had faced and broken the grip of an energy that was both me and not me. I continued to struggle with periodic binges for years after this, but this experience etched itself in my mind, giving me a deep understanding of both the power of samskaras, as well as the possibility of change. Because if you can do it once—break the grip of the samskara, that is—you will more able to do it twice, and then three times, and so on. Once you know you can break the grip, you are also able to right yourself more quickly after a relapse. Please note that my ability to make this break from the samskara did not come out of the blue. I had done a lot of work (therapy, medication, personal growth) that gave me enough strength to dare to pull away from the enticement of its pull. I knew that there was something on the other side of the binge and that I could survive outside the bizarre comfort of the self-destructive samskara.

It is very easy to foreclose in the change process. Rather than seize the moment to effect change, simply solidifying who you are ("addictive," or "fat") or blaming the world is comfortably familiar—and much easier than following through. I like to think of these times when you do manage to hold steady as small, invisible moments of tremendous courage. It's a true victory when through a combination of will, strength, and blind faith, you are able to hold firm in the face of resignation into the old, habitual patterns you have reinforced over a lifetime. As Iyengar states: "Then you build up banks of good nature, bonhomie, openness, nonsmoking, or whatever you want. These form a good character and make our lives much easier."

The concept of samskaras works in both positive and negative directions. Positive actions are self-reinforcing and open up new possibilities for growth and change. Conversely, every limit that is challenged, or defied, in the negative sense opens up new realms of destructive behavior. When I first started bingeing, I remember being surprised that I had eaten seven pieces of toast. Pushing my limits like this triggered a certain giddiness because, on some level, I knew it was "wrong," not in a moral sense, but in the sense of defying an invisible law. The giddiness had to do with the need to stand out or make an imprint, a misguided method of self-assertion. Perhaps it was a "you can't stop me" feeling that egged (and toasted) me on. Then I remember at some later date thinking to myself, "Remember when I thought eating seven pieces of toast was a lot?" Clearly my behavior had escalated. I had habituated to seven pieces, which opened the door to eight, nine, and ten. The same principle applies to any pathological behavior, including drug and ·alcohol use, sexual addiction, and even violence toward others. We flirt with the boundaries of acceptable/unacceptable behavior and, once titillated, we move forward, even at our own peril.

On the positive side of this equation, when I first started running, I remember being very proud of myself when I completed a mile downhill. I was at a country boarding school and in the evening would run and walk from the main campus to my dorm that was about a mile down a tree-lined dirt road. I didn't think I was capable of running a mile, but after a few months, I did it! This was a very pleasurable and, at the time, a deeply private accomplishment. It became private after a male acquaintance had scoffed at my efforts, "You think that will do anything for you?" he demanded, secure in his buff physique. This underlines the need for self-validation, to know what is right for you even when others disagree, or even ridicule. Several months later, I completed three miles and I'll tell you, I was blown away. You'd have thought I had won the Olympics! Years later, running five miles a day was normal, and I could do up to fifteen.

So, by stretching my capacities, my sense of who I was, and what I was capable of, grew. My body and its latent abilities and strength led the way.

Exploring Your Body/Food Samskaras

The way you inhabit your body day to day is a habit of Being. How you breathe, how you walk, and how you feed yourself are habits of Being (samskaras) that invisibly reinforce one another. Changing these ingrained rhythms of self-relationship is possible, but it is gradual. A large portion of your identity, how you define yourself, is wrapped up in how you feed and take care of your body. Self-assessments such as, "I have no willpower," "I am lazy," "I hate exercise," "I'm big boned," are all examples of how you can solidify yourself into a static entity with fixed properties, rather than experiencing yourself as ongoing, unfolding energy that is actually always changing. Aristotle himself put it this way, "We are what we repeatedly do." This is a radical thought because it means that none of us are fixed entities. Although we are products of our past behaviors and thoughts and it is easy to continue to live out these patterns/samskaras, we are also always unfolding and can begin repeating new behavioral patterns. It sounds so easy, doesn't it? The seeming simplicity of this is what motivates you to start a new diet or self-improvement plan—"I'll just do these new things and become new." And we all know how well that works. It is important to have a great deal of respect for the power of samskaras—they go deep. And as mentioned above, patterns of feeding and caring for your body are particularly ingrained. As unhealthy as your patterns might be, you may still feel possessive and have a strong desire to cling to them. "I'm big boned, dammit!" "I have a big appetite!" "But I love food!" Assessing your core beliefs and behavioral patterns around food and your body is an important initial step in the change process. You must make your core beliefs accessible to your conscious scrutiny so you can challenge those that are dysfunctional. This gives you the power to make more conscious choices and opens up the possibility for change.

I am focusing more on common samskaras for women who struggle with feeling too large and out of control with food. The other side of the coin, which is equally painful and destructive, is being overly controlled and restrictive with food. This might sound like, "I don't NEED what others do." "I'm stronger than that." "Carbohydrates are for sissies." In our society, women with this brand of samskara are often admired for their "enviable" self-control and discipline. Underneath the tracks of this samskaras is deep alienation from the flow of life. The need to keep strict controls on her body may look natural from the outside, however, it takes constant vigilance that becomes exhausting over time.

Your body samskaras have **physiological, mental** (thought patterns), **emotional,** and **behavioral** components to them. For example, binge eating has a *physiological track* in your system—perhaps a larger body, less sensitivity to leptin (a hormone signaling satiety), insulin resistance, or a damaged intestinal tract. It has a *mental/cognitive aspect* having to do with your belief system, such as, "I have no self-control" or "My body is inferior/ shameful." The *emotional* component has to do with patterns of helplessness or shame, for example, collapsing into "depression" as a way to foreclose coping responsibly with a problem. The *behavioral aspect* might be related to patterns of eating alone, hoarding food, planning binges, and alternatively starving and gorging. It is always possible to create new positive samskaras, however, to do so you must first increase your awareness of your existing samskaras and their self-reinforcing components.

Reflections on Your Samskaras

1. Think about the physical samskaras that you have created in your body. Imagine how your habits might manifest in your biology. Reflect on your eating habits, your breathing habits, and your movement habits. Patterns of restricted breathing and movement often manifest in an overreliance on food for self-soothing.

2. Can you relate to the energetic aspect of samskaras? If you have a problem with bingeing or feeling out of control with food, reflect upon the energetic aspect of this. Do you ever feel like it's a force that is outside your direct control? Get curious about your experience before overeating: How does it rise in your body? When does it peak? What's it like to fall into the wave? On the other side, if you tend to restrict food, reflect on your associations to hunger and fullness. When do you feel safe and secure in your body?

3. What are some positive samskaras that you have created in your life, either in relation to self-care or something else, like your work or relationships?

4. Reflect on some positive habits/samskaras you would like to develop in relations to self-care.

There is a karmic barrier that you need to break through in the process of change. "Karmic barrier?" This may sound a bit grandiose, but it certainly is relevant to my own experience. There is an energetic field around you that defines who you are and what is possible. It is very easy to stay within the safe confines of this force field (think of the tire tracks in the mud). You feel strong resistance to breaking out of your familiar energetic/behavioral patterns. You resist it because it is feels awkward, unsafe, and uncomfortable … "This isn't right for me," you say to yourself. To which I reply, "Get over yourself!" "Huh?" you might be saying right now, "that doesn't sound very compassionate." But it is, in the sense that I am empathizing with your stuckness and reminding you that the Self you are getting over is just a familiar pattern of thoughts, emotions, and behaviors that you have gotten comfortable with. Yes, these intangibles are also mirrored in the tangible stuff of your body, but this too is amenable to change. In fact, my friend, this is exactly where you need to start off, by addressing the realm of the material, the "stuff" you are made of.

Part Two

A New Perspective on Your Body

Introducing the Kosas

When we think about our body, we typically think of our physical body and most often consider its outward properties—brown hair, medium long, brown eyes, 5-foot-5, large breasts, muscular calves...In yoga philosophy, our physical body, and particularly the outward characteristics of our body, are merely the tip of the iceberg. Yoga identifies five layered bodies moving from the material to increasingly subtle. This perspective is helpful for us as we explore your relationship to food because it deepens your appreciation for your body beyond its looks and size.

Consider a typical day in your life. It's three in the afternoon and you just wrapped up a stressful meeting. You have some paperwork to finish before you go to pick up the kids, get them fed, and send them off to their respective activities. The paperwork is not difficult, but it is tedious and you are feeling...uncomfortable. You are tired from the meeting and don't feel like you have the reserves to put out any more energy. The evening's activities are looming and feel laborious, even though you know that you should be grateful to have two healthy kids and a busy family. Your energy is just so low and you have to get through all those notes and the filing before you have to rush off to get the boys. And you can't help but feel upset by how your boss spoke to you during the meeting. She seems to have been treating you differently ever since you began needing to leave early to get your son to soccer practice. Your mind keeps going back to that comment she made about people managing their hours more responsibly. After all, you have been working there more than five years and have always maintained good output. As these thoughts whirl around in your head, what you may not notice is the tightness in your belly, your jaw, and your shoulders. Or that your breathing is shallow and constricted. What you do notice is that you have a mild headache and you feel very tired. Coffee? No, too jarring and sour on the stomach. Besides, you need to sleep tonight and last night's sleep was a little dicey. You had a lighter meal for lunch because you are trying to lose weight. You are craving something sweet and salty. Pretzels sound like just the thing, though you have been trying to cut back on refined carbohydrates and salt. Oh, that's right, you brought some carrots for a snack. But they just don't sound as good as the pretzels. Yeah, pretzels are the just the thing to get you through the paperwork and into the evening. You can swing by Burger King for the kids and grab a salad there. That will even things out.

You head down the hall to the vending machine, anticipating the salty crunch that is just moments away. The pretzels taste great going down and fill you with a much-needed sense of energy. When you are finished, you want something more. You feel better, but the activities in front of you still feel unpleasant. Some chocolate would really give you the boost you need. You go back to the vending machine for some M&M's. They taste great—the sweet crunch is hypnotizing. You finish the package. Then you feel a familiar rush of guilt. Dammit! Why can't you just have more willpower? You pop a stick of gum in your mouth and get on with your duties.

Let's break down this scenario from the perspective of your different yoga bodies. The tangible, material aspect of your body is called the **annamaya kosa** in yoga philosophy. This includes your outward body, your appearance and physical attributes, as well as your inward body, meaning your viscera, organs, muscles, ligaments, etc. For our purposes, and from a yogic perspective, your outward body is of little concern (as stylish yoga clothes were not around a few thousand years ago). Your inward body, your blood and viscera, however, is far more pertinent from a yogic perspective. In the above scenario, your blood sugar was likely quite low due to your light lunch. Depending on the overall quality of your diet, your organs may not be functioning at an optimal level, possibly impairing your metabolism systemically. Your thyroid, responsible for the proper functioning of every cell in your body, might not be working efficiently, causing you to feel tired and drained. Your cells may be insulin resistant. Insulin is the "key" that allows your cells to accept sugar from your bloodstream and to convert it into energy. When your cells become insulin resistant, they don't accept the sugar, which remains in your bloodstream and damages your tissues. This leaves you physically depleted and also puts strain on your pancreas, which is forced to overproduce insulin to compensate for your cells' difficulty utilizing insulin properly. To add insult to injury, due to your difficult day, your muscles are likely quite tense, constricting the flow of blood and lymph through your body. Your interior system is tired, exhausted from lack of sleep and the demands of your active life. At a physical level, you are just worn out.

The next layer of your Being is your energetic body, which is referred to as the **pranamaya kosa** in yoga philosophy. The energetic layer of your body is the subtle buzz of life that animates you. In yoga, *prana* is life force and is intimately connected to your breath. A whole branch of yoga, called pranayama, is devoted to the regulation of breath/prana. We are energetic beings—our heart has an energetic pulse and our cells communicate energetically. Our ability to regulate our energy efficiently is fundamental to maintaining a healthy body. In the above scenario, your energetic body is depleted and incoherent. There is an element of force rather than a steady rhythm to your energetic body. The idea of "steady rhythm" is best conceptualized as the energy of your heart, which keeps on ticking until it stops. What is the heart's secret? Steady work balanced with rest. Force, on the other hand, is defined as depletion coupled with insistence: "I have to get this work done!" "I have to leave by 4:30 to get the boys!" "But I'm exhausted!" This creates a strong sense of pressure coupled with a very real lack of resources to meet the demands due to your physical body's exhaustion. This situation of high demand coupled with lack of resources is commonly referred to as "stress." Not having the time, or maybe even the knowledge, that some deep breathing could help you, you instead fall back on the samskara (habit) of using food as a quick fix for your energy—and you crave pretzels.

Now your mind, the **manomaya kosa,** the third layer of your body in yoga, steps in. But, alas, your mind is not much help here. Rather, your mind is jangled with worry regarding your boss, the perceived demands of the rest of your day, as well as your desire to lose weight and your "shoulds and shouldn'ts" regarding food choices. The press of your physical body's exhaustion and your energetic body's need for stabilization outweighs any weak commands from your mind to resist the pretzels. The fourth layer of your body, called the **vijnanamaya kosa,** could be of help here. This is your wisdom body, which houses your higher awareness and ability to make choices that are truly in your best interest. Your vague awareness that you "should" be grateful for your healthy, active family is a faint whisper from this layer of your Being. This aspect of your awareness is connected with higher level intelligence that reaches past the needs of the moment and is instead concerned with your greater good. The yogic path aims to help you harness the power of your wisdom body in order to live in a manner consonant with your values and ultimately to obtain greater spiritual awareness.

The ultimate goal of yoga is spiritual awakening. The deepest level of your body is the **anandamaya kosa,** the bliss body. This is the level of universal consciousness, of non-separation with all that is. Non-separation is the deep awareness that we are all interconnected, allowing your individual self to literally melt away in the realization that we are all the same inside. The salutation "Namaste," usually said at the end of a yoga class, is translated as "the light in me sees the light in you." The awareness that astronauts had when he glimpsed the planet Earth from space is a beautiful example of that level of awareness.

The course outlined in this book is not meant to bring you to this higher level of yoga. We will remain firmly grounded in the personal realm of your Being with the intention of utilizing yogic wisdom to enhance your health and self-care. We will touch upon the wisdom body or vijnanamaya kosa in the discussion of developing insight, or the ability to Witness yourself. This capacity represents the interface between your personal consciousness and a larger intelligence to which you begin to avail yourself. Hopefully, through this introduction to yoga, you will begin to touch upon this universal aspect of yourself and your connection to life beyond your individual self. It is here, in the gentle buzzing of your aliveness that you may briefly feel your connection to the aliveness of the universe and allow yourself to be held in this rhythm without need for food, fantasy, or other anchors to buffer your experience.

The following two chapters (chapter 3 and chapter 4) make up part 2 of the book and will explore the annamaya kosa and pranamaya kosa in relation to the yoga of food. This section aims to make this new, yogic understanding of yourself accessible and will give you concrete exercises so that you can apply the ideas to your own life and body.

Chapter Three

Your Physical Body
(Annamaya Kosa)

I briefly had a friend in graduate school who was a much "better" bulimic than I was. She was thinner, sexier, somehow you could tell that she wasn't afraid of bending the rules. I once looked in her refrigerator and saw only a head of broccoli. She captured the imagination. We shared a moment of recognition once, discussing the feeling of waking up the next morning after eating (a lot) the night before, anxiously patting our stomach to see if we "got away with it," meaning, to see if we managed to metabolize the evidence before it lodged itself in bloat and girth. This was a losing battle for me and was always laced with anxiety and a strong sense of impending failure. However, those moments of victory—when the scale reflected the desired number and my regimen of eating, not eating, and exercising evened out to the desired ratio of bone to flesh—made it seem worthwhile. Men would look at me a little longer, women would say enviously, "How do you stay so thin?" These short moments in time were soon lost in spite of my grim efforts. Being the perfect specimen, hitting the right number and the correct size, was not natural to me (or to anyone really), and the game of balancing my hunger and anxiety with appropriate caloric intake exacted its own cost. I had my tricks—lots of gum and candy, skipped meals, daily running, carrots. When I would overeat, my purging method was not eating and exercise until I could work the excesses through my system. It took a toll physically and emotionally.

I tell this little vignette to illustrate the lexicon of the eating disordered. Being a "better" bulimic is obviously not possible. Yet, when I looked at my friend, I imagined that it came more easily for her. I guessed that she didn't suffer from the anxiety or the self-hatred that I did. After all, she was thinner than me. And she looked so cool in her skinny black dress and boots. Maybe I could get it right too … just maybe.

Bulimics play with the laws of nature, while compulsive eaters deny them. You could say that anorexics are attempting to deny nature all together. When you are attempting to outwit the body, to deny or circumvent the laws of nature, you are under the illusion that some people are playing this game "better" than you are. The words of B.K.S. Iyengar put this illusion in a yogic perspective: "The rules of nature cannot be bent. They are impersonal and implacable. But we do play with them. By accepting nature's challenge and joining the game, we find ourselves on a windswept and exciting journey that will pay benefits commensurate to the time and effort we put in …"

This is a very powerful statement when we apply it to your body. Your flesh is tangible and material and functions according to certain rules—universal "rules" regarding food and your body that you may not like very much. So you play with them, try to outwit them, and get around them. This generally leads to more suffering, although it can be fun for a while. These are the moments of "payoff," when you hit the right numbers on the scale or your blood work comes back good in spite of your "bad" behavior. Perhaps you can "get away with it," you think to yourself. And then there are those moments of enjoying a delicious meal with delightful abandon. At times like these, it all seems to work and you see no need to change. More often, however, there is that nagging feeling that all is not well inside. It may show up as, "I really need to take off that ten, twenty, thirty pounds." Or, "I know I need to get a handle on my stress level." These whispers from the inside are what we begin to open to and listen to when we enter the realm of the physical body/annamaya kosa.

Yoga is a process by which you begin to learn about and integrate the laws of nature as they apply to your body. Remember, *yoga* means "to yoke" or "unite." You begin to yoke your external knowledge of how to care for your body with your internal sense of what is good for you. At its most basic level, the yoga of food means recognizing that some foods and habits serve you better than other foods and habits. At a slightly more elevated level, it means honoring your body's internal feedback system and letting your body accept that feedback, rather than allowing external rules to guide your self-care/food choices. Essentially, the yoga of food is about integrating what you know about the "rules" of nature as they apply to your body, and living in accordance with these rules. As you progress along the path of yoga, it becomes less about manipulating your body to be a particular way (thin or healthy), and more about appreciating your body as an expression of universal intelligence.

Get Under Your Skin

My client Moxie has been through the wars. Diagnosed with aggressive breast cancer at thirty-six and positive for the BRCA gene (a mutation linked with high likelihood of breast and ovarian cancer), she has endured radical double mastectomy and hysterectomy procedures. Then, after having her gallbladder removed, she subsequently had her entire colon, anus, and rectum removed due to an early stage diagnosis of colon cancer.

Despite these setbacks, she maintains a no-nonsense approach to life and is determined to see her child through his youth. Sporting a blond pixie haircut and a forthright manner, she is the kind of gal you know would do anything to protect the ones she loves. Why is it then that she can't love herself? And why does she keep sabotaging her health with afternoon junk food and evening ice cream? "I feel like a marshmallow with a pinhead," she declares with her usual self-deprecating laugh. She describes working out in the gym and feeling pretty good afterward. This positive reconnection with her body is then swept away by regret when she catches a glimpse of herself in the mirror. She is well aware of her body dysmorphia, "I feel mutilated," she declares, without self-pity, knowing that these habits of denigrating her body preceded her cancer diagnoses. The work for Moxie, as for many of us, is to learn to see herself beyond the apologetic image in the mirror and beyond the glare of what is wrong with, or missing from, her body. This is deep work, particularly for Moxie, having so suddenly (within seven years) been forced to endure the loss of her youthful, pristine body. We discuss the importance of learning to put her health first, to not "flake" on herself, but to use her precious energy to enhance her own well-being. I talk to her about the need to delve beneath her fixation on her appearance and bring a new commitment to life under her skin.

Moving Inside

Shift your perspective away from your own body for a moment and think about what a marvelous entity you are. You are a self-contained, finely calibrated system. You can stand on your head and your body knows what to do to equalize pressure and hold your vital organs in place. Your heart beats away, pumping blood where it needs to go, oxygenating your tissues and your brain. You decide to move your toes and voilà, you move your toes. When your body tells you to hydrate, you get something to drink. If only eating when you are hungry was such a simple process!

In our culture we are mesmerized by externals—the size of your hips and thighs, the wrinkles and gray hair—and it is so pervasive that it eclipses your attention so you don't notice what is going on under your skin, right under your nose, so to speak. Rather than marveling in the complexity and ingenuity of your physical self, you may perpetuate a contentious, critical relationship with your body. It becomes habitual to focus on what is not going well, nitpicking the imperfections, comparing your body to other, seemingly better models. This creates an internal rift, a dissonance that can disrupt your ability to appreciate your body, let alone your life. A shift in perspective is necessary to take a peek inside and develop more gratitude for what is happening just beneath your skin. You might say that in our culture, most of us suffer from an extreme lack of imagination. This is the meaning of the word "ignore-ance"—think of this as a verb indicating the act of ignoring what is. In Iyengar's words, "It is an obsession in our modern society to focus on appearance, presentation, and packaging. We do not ask ourselves, 'How am I really?' but 'How do I look, how do others see me?' It is not a question of 'What am I saying?' but 'How do I sound?'" So captivated by the appearance and grooming of our flesh, we are blind to the magic and complexity of our physical beings. This means appreciating what is going right with your body. If you are alive, there is more going right than wrong. It also means developing some concern about unnecessary strain your daily habits may be perpetuating. The decline in energy and well-being that many of us experience as we age is gradual, so it is easy to ascribe subtle symptoms to the inevitable slowing down of aging. Unless you have some sort of obvious problem, like cancer or chronic fatigue, you may underestimate the burden that your body is under. Your body tends to make the best of things until the proverbial straw breaks the camel's back. This discussion of your internal health is not meant to be alarmist or preachy. It is meant to give you more awareness of the fact that your body is real, it is subject to the laws of nature, and your insides are as real as the your outside.

As you read on, I want you to be aware of your internal reaction. Do you start to get anxious as you think about your insides? Do you begin to dissociate a bit, perhaps skimming the text with less attention? Do you get overwhelmed? Your reactions are all grist for the mill. Assimilate what you can and trust your own process. You are reading this, after all, which in and of itself signifies some new awareness and growth. Remember, you don't have to do everything at once. You can change your habits slowly and respectfully over time.

So let us turn now to your digestive tract. Yes, that slippery tube inside you from mouth to anus. As you know, you are dependent upon food as an energy source to keep your body alive and to provide the nutrients that allow for the ongoing functioning of your body's various systems. Your digestive tract assimilates these nutrients. The system works like this—you choose foods with various nutritional components and chew them up in your mouth to begin the digestive process. Saliva is a magic substance that rushes in to help break down your food and kill bacteria. You then swallow the food so that it can travel to your stomach, where it mixes up with more digestive juices and a small amount of hydrochloric acid to further break down the food, kill bacteria, and release nutrients for absorption. This slurry (called chyme) is then transported through your small and large intestines, where nutrients are gradually absorbed and delivered to the rest of your body. The components of the foods that are not used travel into the lower colon and out your body. All of this is in the service of fueling your body for ongoing life.

We all know that we need to eat to live and that our digestive tracts are designed to process the foods we take in. But, even though you "know" this in your head, if you have food issues, you likely eat with very little attention to the needs of your body. You may choose foods based on caloric content, or the latest nutritional advice (if you are being "good"), and perhaps consume whatever/whenever in a dissociated frenzy (when you are being "bad"). During a "good" phase, you may choose heavily processed, artificially engineered materials designed to supposedly help you lose weight. You may give little thought to the impact these substances have on the vital processes occurring under your skin. The other side of this coin is consuming the heavily flavored, sugared substances designed by our food industry to excite and stimulate your appetite. The two habits go hand in hand—restrictive, calculated ingestion of what you "should" eat with the goal to get yourself under control followed by a free-for-all that reliably comes as an inevitable response to deprivation.

At a less extreme level, perhaps you have more consistent eating habits but rarely stop to consider the food's quality and the impact of what you are consuming has on your vital system. Your eating habits are so routine and utilitarian that almost no attention is paid to quality or quantity—and even less attention goes toward enjoyment, taking pleasure in a meal. On the flip side are those of you who do not eat enough, who thrive on deprivation and the challenge of seeing how little you can get by on. If you suffer from any of the above habits, it is important to not criticize or disparage yourself. Your relationship with food and your body is just that, a relationship. As I have mentioned, yoga is commonly defined as "union," or "to yoke." The yoga of food is based on healing your relationship with food and your body. Feeling into your insides and learning to hold yourself with reverence, as opposed to either controlling or indulging yourself, is the common path of healing for us all.

Due to the content of our modern diet and the process of our modern lifestyle (rush, rush, rush, worry, worry, worry), the internal lining of the digestive tract can become inflamed, which interferes with your ability to digest and assimilate food. This can lead to food intolerances, which though not as severe as allergies, will create a cycle of instability in your system. When you are unwittingly perpetuating this cycle with what you eat, you have very little power to change—mainly because you are unaware that anything is amiss. As I said, when you are focused on externals, the cosmetics of the situation, you overlook the reality underlying the condition of your body. Healing from the inside out is both frightening and empowering. It is frightening because it can shatter some of your denial (your "ignore-ance"). If you are under the impression that you just need to "lose a few pounds," or that you are "a little run-down," it can be quite a game changer to realize that the fuel you have been providing (or not providing!) your body is a cause that has left an effect inside. This is a wake-up call, an "uh-oh" moment. It can also be very empowering. By facing the reality of what is going on beneath your skin, which takes courage and a paradigm shift (you are looking inside now, rather than being mesmerized by your image), you have the power to take charge in a new way. There are things that you can do to address the health of your insides. You can learn to choose foods with more awareness regarding how they affect your body. You can begin to feel what is good for you as your awareness begins to expand beneath your skin. As you make wiser choices and develop more care and appreciation for your body, you also start to feel better. This is the sweetest outcome of all. You get more in touch with your capacity for pleasure and well-being, rather than dependent upon food substances that do little good for your body.

In order to heal your relationship with food, it is essential that you bring attention and appreciation to the world beneath your skin and learn to honor your body. The paradigm shift I refer to above is not really a "moment," but rather a process of unlearning old habits of thinking about your body and food. It certainly does not mean that you must forsake pleasure in eating or that you must deprive yourself of good things. It means learning to expand your idea of pleasure to enjoying the pleasure of a well-nourished, healthy body. Think of this process as additive rather than depriving. "What can I add to my repertoire of foods and activities that will encourage trust and confidence in my body?" The journey for all of us is allowing this enjoyment to become more embodied, meaning eating food is an act of appreciation for the nourishment the food is providing, rather than a compulsive, dissociated activity that ends up being abusive toward your body.

Reflections on Your Body

1. Consider what is going well in your body at this moment. Perhaps you have good knees. Do you have a strong heart? A hearty digestive system? Perhaps you don't have a headache. If you're anything like me, you don't stop to appreciate what feels good, and instead your attention is captured by the ache, pain and imperfection.

2. When is the last time that you went to the doctor for a checkup? I thought so. Make an appointment with your primary care doctor to get a basic blood panel, including cholesterol, triglycerides, thyroid, iron, blood sugar, and any other tests that you and your doctor deems relevant. You will likely resist doing this. I know I do. However, it is important to get a concrete sense of how your body is doing as you seek to take charge of your health in a more proactive way.

3. You might consider consulting a naturopathic doctor to assess the health of your digestive tract. This is especially relevant if you suffer from low energy or digestive problems. A naturopath can give you advice regarding healing your digestive tract and accelerate your course toward improved health. I suggest you seek out someone who has gone to an accredited school and is licensed to practice naturopathy.

The Karma of Food

The idea of karma is a widely known and accepted concept in our society. Our interpretation of it here in the West is quite different than its meaning in Classical Yoga, which deems karma an undesirable force that holds us to unending incarnations. For our purposes, I am going to stick to the Western meaning, which highlights the relationship between cause and effect. Every action has a reaction, or ripple effect. Although the concept of karma as we interpret it here in the West is not foolproof—after all, bad things happen to good people all the time—more often than not this simple formula has its utility because it helps us stay accountable to our actions. You may be familiar with the saying "what goes around, comes around." When discussing food, we could rephrase the formula as the ubiquitous "you are what you eat." Food matters. It is matter that contains energy that has an effect on your body. As Iyengar states, "When we eat a head of lettuce, every leaf expresses the beauty and complexity of the cosmic intelligence that formed it, and so we are partaking of cosmic intelligence by ingesting it directly."

I recently had a conversation with a client who was in the habit of having chips and soda for breakfast. "Would you put low-grade gas in a high-performance car?" I asked her. "Well, of course not," she replied, recognition subtly lighting in her eyes. I pressed on, "And why not?" "Because it wouldn't run as well and over time it would degrade and start to have problems."

Exactly. I am not suggesting that you should think of yourself as a high-performance car, as this is rather objectifying. But I do suggest that you consider whether you treat your car better than your body (which, after all, you cannot trade in when it wears out), and if you do, pause for a moment to reflect on this.

Not only is it true that "you are what you eat," taking it a step further we could add, "you are what you assimilate." I once heard it explained this way: our bodies are like computers and the food we put into them contains certain information that our bodies are designed to read. Your body knows how to read the information contained within fruits, vegetables, and other whole foods. Throw in the hydrogenated fats and high-fructose corn syrup and you've got a programming mess—your body doesn't know how to read the information, leading to our larger societal problems of skyrocketing rates of type 2 diabetes and heart disease. The truth is that whole foods from the earth are best for us. Spinach, carrots, lentils … As an aside, though you may think of lentils, spinach, and others of their ilk as supremely unpalatable, I hope to convince you otherwise later on.

The type of food you put into your body is a "cause" that will bring about a particular "effect" in your body. What you choose to eat matters. The laws of karma apply. For most of us (though not Moxie, who bears a genetic burden making her more vulnerable to disease), we can "get away with it," meaning we have the dubious luxury of neglecting our health to a degree, when we are young. Around forty years or so, bad habits begin to knock at the door to collect. You are more tired, labs aren't so good, and some of you get more scary diagnoses that shake your invulnerability. Genetics play a huge role in what you can get away with and when and how your lifestyle habits will collect. Some of you will get cancer, diabetes, or an autoimmune disorder in spite of a healthy lifestyle. And then there is the opposite extreme, embodied by Keith Richards, the guitarist for the Rolling Stones, who God love him, should be dead from multiple causes by now. No matter what your health status, the line from the movie *Unforgiven,* when Clint Eastwood tells his young, cocky companion in his classic deadpan tone, "Kid, we all got it comin'..." has great relevance for all of us with regard to our health. The realization that, sorry to say, "you got it coming" in some form or other can serve as a powerful impetus to do what you can to take care of yourself today by making more mindful decisions regarding what kind of "causes" you want to apply in your daily life. Being a more mindful custodian of your body will pay great dividends in your present life and your future well-being, regardless of your current weight or health status.

Applying the concept of karma to food/weight issues entails cultivating an acceptance of your body as a representation, a result, of past behaviors. Your body is a conglomeration of your genetics and your past behaviors and beliefs about health. This is not a permanent condition, however, you must contend with it directly in order to initiate change. Meeting your body in the here and now means not focusing on your present condition in a disparaging way (as in, "my thighs are so fat!") or focusing on the size or weight that you must be in a month or next year ("I have to lose weight for the wedding!"). Rather, it is a commitment to steering your flesh in a different direction, one that is aligned with better health and well-being. This is an act of faith because it requires leaping beyond the present state of affairs and trusting that different behaviors over time will create different circumstances. Most of us go awry by over focusing on results, on the visible "realities." You need lower numbers on the scale, a smaller clothes size, or your commitment derails. You leave the gym after a good workout and are flummoxed by the image in the mirror.

Your taste—that is, the foods you gravitate toward—are also a product of your past behaviors and conditioning. You likely associate certain foods with comfort, health, and normalcy, often with very little information. My husband, for example, was confounded when we watched the movie *Super Size Me* and learned just how unhealthy ice cream is due to its saturated fat content. "I always thought ice cream was wholesome," he said in a regretful tone, another illusion of childhood gone. Isn't this exactly what commercials appeal to—our tendency to lump arbitrary associations in our mind without discrimination? It is important to begin challenging some of your conditioned associations. Do you see salads as depriving, unappealing, or for sissies? Is a big steak "healthy" because it helps you build muscle? Are people who eat healthfully strange or puritanical? Are lentils or spinach an unpalatable consolation prize or potentially delicious sustenance for your mind and body?

If you are in the habit of relying on food to satisfy needs other than nourishment, you are set up for difficulty. As I have mentioned, food can be a lovely feature of living in a body on this planet. However, it is a bonus, not the main feature. If you have been using it as the main feature, or if you use it to support the main feature in a dysfunctional way (as in, "Let me get through this heinous meeting, activity, function, so I can go eat"), then physical satisfaction is something that you will need to re-find. This gets complicated because, according to the laws of karma (action-reaction), your body has become habituated to particular ways of eating, which have created conditions in your body that you now must contend with. For example, leptin and ghrelin are hormones related to satiety and hunger respectively. When you have been eating high-sugar/high-fat, low-nutrient food for many years, these hormones are not going to be working in your favor. Meaning, you are not going to be sensitive to leptin, which signals when you are full, and your ghrelin may function as a ravenous little gremlin, signaling hunger all the time. Thus, hormonally you are in a bit of a pickle. (If only a pickle was all that you were craving!) On the flip side, someone who has anorexic patterns may have more ghrelin circulating in her system and yet she has habituated herself not to respond to it—she is ghrelin-resistant. This is a poignant example of how the will can be used to subvert the natural signals of the body. The challenge is learning not to respond habitually to your "hunger"/or lack thereof, but to gently guide your physiology away from what feels "good" (or familiar) in the immediate sense to what feels better in a long-term sense. Satisfaction may change from the heavy feeling after a rich, high-carbohydrate meal to the lighter feeling after a large salad with protein. Or the peace felt by restricting food and being lightheaded and empty can shift to the peace of knowing that you are caring for your body by allowing yourself to accept nourishment. Either change will be highly uncomfortable at first because it is outside the habituated pattern. You might interpret your lack of fullness as "hunger" if you are used to being heavily anchored to the earth by food. Or you might feel "stuffed/fat" if you are used to a constant state of emptiness. Learning to interpret either side of the discomfort as anxiety wrought from change rather than as hunger that needs to be quenched, or fullness that needs to be eradicated, is a huge step in learning to relate to food in a more sane, holistic way.

———

Sophie, a twenty-two-year-old woman whom you shall hear more about later on, recently shared with me that when she wants to eat when she is not hungry, she is learning to just "sit with" the uncomfortable feeling. She has been largely abandoned by her parents, who are now going through an ugly divorce. Her father is living somewhere else, unable to help her financially, and rarely contacts her. Her mother is involved in a new relationship and is pressuring Sophie to get a job so she can move out. No one seems to consider that this might be an inappropriate expectation given that Sophie has extreme social anxiety, which is why she was allowed to leave high school when she was fifteen. She is bravely trying to face up to the task of growth, but at times she feels overwhelmed, particularly when she is home alone and has free access to the ready comfort of food. "I am learning to just stay with the anxiety," she said to me recently, "and I am learning that the anxiety passes," she elaborated, "but it is soooo uncomfortable." Another client shared with me her experience of feeling compelled to binge on fast food but knowing that "just this once," wasn't going to cut it anymore. She lay on her bed repeating to herself, "It's just tire tracks in my mind. It's just tire tracks in my body. It's possible to create new ones." What courage and fortitude it takes for these young women to sit in the nameless waves of such consuming hungers without filling them with food. It helps to remember that the feelings will pass, as well as the fact that you are not alone in having them.

So here is the challenge. You commit to meeting "what is," meaning the current condition of your body, with the intention to act in the best interest of your body even if it is uncomfortable in the moment. The leap of faith is trusting that over time, what is good for you will begin to appeal to you more and more. At the beginning, rather than focusing on your weight (numbers, after all, can be deceiving), I suggest tracking the effect that different foods have on your sense of well-being, your energy levels, and the pattern of your hunger. I also suggest using your mind (manomaya kosa) to guide your choices. This is where mind can be helpful. Research the foods that health experts suggest. Make decisions about what to eat based upon what you know about nutrition. Many women with weight issues are veritable encyclopedias regarding calories and health. The necessary shift is to transform this information into knowledge, that is, into a knowing that is embodied and lived. The attitude that you will need to cultivate is patience with the process, shifting focus from "results" (such as losing weight) and trusting that over time what feels unfamiliar or depriving will become more natural. Also trust that this process is not about self-deprivation, but is about learning to align what you want with what is good for you. This is a worthwhile endeavor for many reasons. It reduces the amount of energy you needlessly expend in neurotic conflict (the "I want it!" "You shouldn't have it!" argument inside), freeing this energy so that it is available for more meaningful pursuits. It also provides you with a deeper feeling of satisfaction—

what you want is actually good for you. Imagine that! As Iyengar puts it, "People forget that in our quest for the soul, we first reclaim the pristine joys of the animal kingdom, health and instinct, vibrant and alive."

Homework for Understanding Your Eating Habits

1. Start keeping a food journal. You may resist this because eating "should" be natural and you rebel against putting so much time into thinking about it. Or perhaps it is because of the accountability a food journal brings to your habitual patterns. Or the ubiquitous "It's boring." "I don't have time." In order to change, you have to have a good sense of what you need to change—and a food journal gives you exactly that. I suggest tracking your mood and energy levels along with what you are eating. This will help you piece together patterns around what you are eating and how you are feeling.

2. Take some time to reflect on your overall eating habits. How much of your daily repast is processed, amalgamated food products vs. actual whole foods? What aspects of your eating habits are healthful? Now list some changes that you would like to make, perhaps cooking more, eating more salads or fresh fruit, or reducing portion size.

3. How much faith do you have that small changes over time will lead in a direction of positive change? What strategies will you use to support yourself when you are feeling discouraged? Support groups, journaling, reading inspirational literature, and nature are all examples of supports that can open up your perspective from hopelessness to openness.

Learning a New Way

Janice initiated therapy with me after months of acute depression that she had been trying mightily to cope with on her own. She is a bright, hard-working person who takes her responsibilities to her friends and her job very seriously. She is no stranger to self-sacrifice and her depression was one more thing she thought she should just be able to plow through. Her efforts had not been successful. One of Janice's main issues is that she cares for others far better than she does for herself. She has wept in my office over the death of her good friend's infant son subsequent to having spent many days at the hospital supporting her grieving friend. She has a harder time acknowledging her own pain, which she tends to minimize and rationalize, "Oh, it wasn't that bad." Over the months of her weekly therapy sessions, she began to agree with me that it was "that bad."

When Janice became valedictorian of her high school, her father commented, "I don't care if you get a PhD in prostitution, you're getting a PhD." His words still ring in her ears twenty years later. Other memories gradually emerge and are woven through our weekly sessions. Being forced in the fourth grade to finish food she did not want until she vomited at the dinner table. The mandated workouts in the eighth grade in front of her father, who commanded her to continue from his armchair. After these humiliating sessions, she would retreat into her bedroom and binge on her hidden stash of junk food, which at the time served as her only form of self-assertion. Then there was the time in high school when her mother didn't speak to her for a month after hearing Janice make a snarky comment about her to a friend. In desperation, Janice begged her mother to forgive her, but she was stone. And these are just the family memories.

There was the doctor that she worked for at sixteen who repeatedly chased her around the exam table to cop a feel. Oh yes, and that adolescent cousin who French kissed her when she was under five years old. Her parents fluffed it off when she told them, and allowed her to continue to share a bedroom with him.

I have commented to Janice that I am surprised, given the emotional trauma of her background, that she does not have more serious mental health and personality problems. We agree that food served as her anchor, gave her that thing to hold on to, that way to rebel, affirm, and comfort herself in the midst of unpredictable and sometimes sadistic behavior. Her use of food to punish herself is a new realization. The memory that marks the genesis of her distorted relationship with food started out innocently enough. At a family gathering celebrating her father's birthday, five-year-old Janice accidentally poured too much Hershey's syrup on her ice cream. Her enraged father forced her to pour the whole can of syrup into her bowl and eat it. The adults, including her mother, stood by. Janice says that on some level she knew that her father's behavior was wrong. However, it was far safer to turn the anger inside, where it morphed into self-hatred expressed by self-abuse with food for the following thirty years. The fact that she has also used food for comfort and anchoring only serves to illustrate the complexities of the human heart and palate.

Janice now weighs more than three hundred pounds. Her dawning recognition of her self-hatred and use of food to punish herself has been startling. "When I get fast food, I only give my dog little bites because I know it's bad for him." She says this incredulously, stupefied by the fact that she treats her dog better than she treats herself.

Janice is currently learning how to eat. She grew up with no real meal times. People in her family ate when and what they wanted from the cupboards and refrigerator stocked with American cheese, white bread, hot dogs, pizza, and chips. Learning how to eat real food is painstaking, both because of the intense emotional aspects of coming to terms with childhood abuse, but also the behavioral and physiological aspects of retraining a mind and body used to consuming large quantities of highly processed foods. She is faced with the challenge of employing restraint without triggering the violent hunger, fueled by entitlement, rage and despair, hovering just below the surface. Janice initially went on a medically supervised weight-loss program but decided after losing sixty pounds that she did not want to consume the artificially flavored, nutrified substance advocated by the program. "I want to learn how to eat real food," she told me. Now she is experimenting with vegetables and cooking. She is slowly, through trial and error, becoming more familiar with her patterns and her pitfalls. "I realize that I cannot have processed foods in the house," she declared after consuming a box of Fiber One bars in one sitting. She also realizes that although her choices are getting better—she's eating real food after all—she cannot eat a pound of pasta for dinner, even if it is whole wheat.

Let us join Janice on her journey of learning how to eat real food in appropriate portions. Remember the laws of karma and let food begin to matter to you in a different way. You can begin to approach food as matter that is here for your enjoyment, as well as for the nourishment of your mind, body, and soul.

Janice is not alone in her struggle to eat more nutritiously. Most of us here in the United States eat the Standard American Diet, or SAD. This acronym was coined in the 1970s as awareness of the poor quality of the typical American's diet was increasingly recognized. The SAD consists of de-nutritionalized grains, amalgamated fats and sugars, chemical additives, and mass-produced, hormone- and antibiotic-injected (some would say tormented) animal protein. Because most of us grew up eating this way, we are conditioned to believe that it is "normal" and don't even give it a second thought—ice cream is "wholesome" after all.

But if you don't question the stuff you are fueling yourself with, you instead end up berating yourself for being "fat" and bemoaning your sluggish metabolism. While metabolism certainly plays a role, hating yourself for a biological trait you've inherited does not accomplish anything. Perhaps it is time to be proactive and question your conditioning regarding what is appropriate fare for your body.

There is so much conflicting nutritional advice out there. Who hasn't been confused by the "fact" that eggs are the devil one day and healthy the next? Dairy is deadly, or it helps you lose weight? Meat has a bad name. But then in the next breath we are told to eat lean proteins and fewer carbs. Coffee? It fights diabetes or contains a drug we should avoid? Wine? Good for the heart or poison for the organs? What you read depends upon the day. What I am struck by is the compartmentalization of "facts" that drives our health information. I receive the Tufts Newsletter, which publishes scientifically based research on nutrition. They may do a study on vitamin D and run scientifically controlled experiments to determine the health effects of this supplement. But, in the end, at least for me, it becomes meaningless. Because, can you really extract one nutritional element and then study its effects in isolation? The synergy of human health is far more complex than that. I am reminded of the parable of three blind men trying to describe an elephant after feeling three different locations of the elephants' body. Yes, they successfully describe the part they are exposed to (the trunk, the legs, and the tail), but they do nothing to approach a meaningful understanding of the whole elephant. The other thing that such compartmentalized advice overlooks is your own internal wisdom regarding what is right for you, what your body needs, and what feels good in an intuitive way. Iyengar states, "Instinct is the unconscious intelligence of the cells surfacing." Information that is dissociated from your instinct does nothing to reestablish your basic sense of trust in yourself and your ability to determine what is good for you.

The best, most succinct, and noncontradictory nutritional advice I have heard is from Michael Pollan, author of *The Omnivore's Dilemma* and *In Defense of Food.* His motto: "Eat food. Not too much. Mostly plants." I love this advice because it is nonpunitive and it isn't rigid and full of magic promises ("Eat dairy, lose weight!"). The following sections will break down this deceptively simple advice and add a little "scientific" data that I have gathered over the years. I put the word scientific in quotes because it seems to me that when it comes to the subject of nutrition and human health you can find a study, or at least an opinion, to back up any "fact" that you want to be true. So, let's try to find some common sense here amidst the deluge of foods and facts facing us today.

The yoga of food asks us to bring together our internal knowledge about what is good for us with our behavior, meaning we unite intention with action. You have to trust yourself, even when you don't "know" what you are doing. In other words, allow yourself to be a beginner and make mistakes while learning something new. This is similar to when you go through a yoga flow when you don't really know what you are doing, but then after a few moves you enter the practice in spite of yourself. It is an act of faith to begin, but you have to start somewhere. So step to the front of your mat and take a breath.

Eat Food

"Eat food." You may be saying, "Duh, that's my problem, I eat too much of it." We'll get to that later. If your struggle is more the anorexic/ orthorexic mentality, you may find yourself recoiling. After all, your main focus has been avoiding eating food. So let's hear Mr. Pollan out and try to assimilate what he means by this simple two-word sentence? In his book *In Defense of Food*, he recommends that we don't eat anything that our grandmothers would not recognize as food from their dinner tables. He discusses the fact that our grocery stores are filled with food substances, meaning various conglomerations of wheat, corn, fat, sugar, and chemical components to make it all tasty. Our grandmothers would likely be befuddled by the long list of chemical ingredients on the labels.

So then, what is food? Food is material derived from the earth that we can use to fuel our bodies. The less processed the better. This is not a moralistic, self-denying position. It's really just common sense. What happens when we primarily dine on highly processed, adulterated food substances? Let's look at the humble pretzel, a simple little snack consisting of processed white flour, oil, a little sugar or high-fructose corn syrup, and a hefty punch of sodium. A great afternoon snack, right, given that it is not fried or particularly sweet? Well, not so much.

When you eat high-sugar food or simple carbohydrates—like pretzels, like many processed cereals and all fruit juices, your body gets a quick hit of glucose in the bloodstream. Your body responds to this surge of glucose by pumping out insulin to neutralize the circulating sugar. This brings your blood sugar down within an hour or two, but it can bring it too far down, resulting in your weak, depleted, "hungry" feeling. So, although you are experientially "ravenous," you probably are not calorie deprived—you just need a sugar fix to bring your flagging blood sugar back up to normal. You can see how this leads to an unhealthy roller coaster of simultaneous overconsumption of calories and nutritional depletion. Aside from the short-term negative effects of riding the blood sugar roller coaster (weight gain, low energy), there are serious long-term effects including insulin resistance (your cells become less sensitive to insulin and require more to respond), which over the long haul can lead to type 2 diabetes. Also, the empty calories waste an opportunity to bring in foods that actually help your body in its daily travails.

The key to addressing this problem is to "eat food." Whole food. Even high-carbohydrate foods, like beans, fruit, and brown rice are beneficial for blood sugar control. This is because they come with copious amounts of fiber, which slows the absorption of sugar into your bloodstream. Nature has some nifty packaging. Consequently, your body does not have to pump out as much insulin so quickly to stabilize your blood sugar. You stay fuller longer because your body is fueled slowly over time, rather than via a quick, short-acting surge of sugar. Another benefit is that all these food contain lots of antioxidants and nutrients, and many, such as beans and quinoa, contain protein as well.

It is actually not too hard, and can be very satisfying, to eat in a blood-sugar friendly way. I have always had a problem processing carbs and discovered in my thirties that the ubiquitous pretzel, much as I loved the salty crunch, did me no favors in the mood or energy department two hours later. Switching over to nuts, vegetables with some dressing, or cheese is not too difficult and is quite delicious. Whole-wheat pasta with pesto or with vegetables and a little cheese is quite a treat at dinner. Salads can be occasions for creativity and celebration when given a little time, good dressing, and thoughtful extras like roasted vegetables, artichoke hearts, or beets. Bean dishes can be prepared from scratch without too much fuss and are a far cry from the canned refried beans you might be used to. The idea here is to slowly introduce whole-grain pastas, sweet potatoes, root vegetables, and other fruits of the earth mixed with spices and good fats to make blood-sugar, body-friendly meals that will feel as good going down as they will make you feel in two hours. Some other blood-sugar friendly ideas include adding acids, such as vinegar or lemon to your meals, which slows the breakdown of starches into sugar. In addition, common spices, such as cinnamon and turmeric, seem to stabilize blood sugar. Turmeric has anti-inflammatory properties, as well as possibly fighting cancer.

The next category of "food" that deserves a word or two is fat. Yes, fat. If ever there was a food category that has been maligned one day and hailed as a savior the next, it is fat. The important thing about fat is the kind you eat. There are some real bad guys in the fat department but luckily there are some real good guys as well. Usually I am not an advocate of black and white thinking. However, when it comes to fat, I am willing to jump on the bandwagon and vilify some of the substances that have made it into our food supply.

The worst of the "bad guys" are the non-food substances that are inserted into prepackaged and fast foods. These fats are dangerous to consume even occasionally. They are **transfats** and their newest permutation, **interestified** fats. Transfats are found in the partially or fully hydrogenated vegetable oils that are used in commercially processed foods in part because they extend the shelf life. However, some restaurants have actually banned the use of transfats because of their clear implication in heart disease. Interestified fats are the food industry's response. These come under the names interestified soybean/vegetable oil and partially or fully hydrogenated oil or stearic acid. Being a relatively new concoction, there is no clear link between interestified fats and heart disease. That's not to say they do not have any health implications. Not only do these fats raise LDL and lower HDL (by the way, H is for "happy," it's the good cholesterol), they also appear to raise blood sugar and depress insulin levels. This raises the risk of developing type 2 diabetes, which is on the rise in our nation.

The yoga of food asks you to consider the impact that foods are having on the inside and to cultivate your intuitive wisdom regarding what is good for you. This takes time to develop, as you may feel quite "good" after eating something "bad" for you. Yoga asks you to try new things (in this case, foods rather than a body position) and work with the initial discomfort before writing it off. So what are the good fats? Here are some suggestions. Omega-3 fats are the fats found in fish, abundantly in salmon, sardines, and anchovies. Plant sources include flaxseeds and walnuts. These foods, and particularly fish, are excellent sources of EFAs, essential fatty acids. They are referred to as "essential" because they are necessary for human health and the body is unable to produce them on its own. EFAs perform vital functions such as lowering triglycerides, lowering LDL (the "bad" cholesterol) and aiding in proper functioning of the metabolism, including insulin regulation. They are also essential for proper brain function. Omega-6s, which are also EFAs, are beneficial fats as well. They are found in nuts, seeds, and olive oil. Olive oil is a monounsaturated fat, rich in omega-6s, that has numerous health benefits, including lowering circulating cholesterol and decreasing inflammation. So consider replacing your bottled fat-free salad dressing and chop up a garlic clove and mix a cup of olive oil with a half cup of vinegar. You may resist this because it seems time-consuming or messy, but try it anyway and see if you like it. One more note, although omega-6s are beneficial, it is important to have a proper ratio of omega-6s to omega-3s. The proper ratio is thought to be 3 to 1 (omega-6s to omega-3s). Most of us do not eat enough fish, walnuts, and flax to approximate this healthy ratio. You can add walnuts to salads, buy canned wild salmon, and grind up a tablespoon of flaxseeds (just use a coffee grinder) for your cereal or yogurt.

The more common "bad" fats are the saturated fats found in red meats and dairy, such as butter, cream, and egg yolks. Occasional, moderate intake of these fats is fine. Overconsumption has been thought to be dangerous due to their negative effect on cholesterol. Recent research has revealed that these fats may not increase cholesterol, but rather it is inflammation in the body (caused by transfats and their ilk) that causes cholesterol to increase. I think the upshot of the issue is that moderation, not deprivation, makes the most sense in your approach to these foods.

So, in this new pursuit of eating real food, gradually introduce fresh, whole foods into your diet. This does take more planning and preparation, but I think you will also be tickled by how delicious this food is. And there is something that feels really good when you eat food that is colorful and flavorful—your body knows that it is good for you and this actually increases your enjoyment. Pleasure that is integrated, rather than dissociated from your body, is the goal of this new, "old" way of eating. A client who struggles with food restriction recently shared with me that she now asks herself when she wants to restrict, "Is this good for me?" She is learning to listen to her body and to make choices to eat or not eat that are integrated with her body's needs rather than her predetermined decision. That's the yoga of food!

Mostly Plants

I'll save the contentious "not too much" part of the formula for later. First, let's talk about plants. And no, Michael Pollan is not asking you to be a vegetarian. Why plants? And what does he even mean by plants? Plants, in my reading of his message, refers to anything that is grown from the earth, including lettuce, carrots, beets, celery, potatoes, whole grains like oats, quinoa, whole wheat, and fruits, which although technically are the fruit of plants, I'll take the liberty of including here. There are at least three important reasons to make the majority of your food intake plants.

Fiber. In some health books that I have read, I have come across the phrase, "Death starts in the colon." To add to this drama and morbidity, I have received health publications (yes, I am on some bizarre mailing lists) that claim that John Wayne, poor soul, had forty pounds of fecal matter in his colon at the time of his death. I recently googled this and the topic does come up, but it appears to be bunk. It just shows how hysterical we can become. All drama and hyperbole aside, there is some truth to be found here, if not regarding the impacted fecal matter in John Wayne's colon, at least in regard to the importance of having regular bowel movements. In order to be healthy, you must be able to release waste from your body. To do so, your body requires sufficient fiber. Eating the whole foods way—incorporating plants in copious quantities to your diet—will make a big difference. Standard recommendations suggest that you get 25 to 30 grams of fiber a day, however, many alternative health practitioners advocate even more. I recommend building up your intake slowly so as not to shock your system if you are not used to eating a lot of fiber. Fiber comes in two main categories, soluble and insoluble. Soluble fibers dissolve, attract water and slow down digestion, which can help stabilize blood sugar levels. Insoluble fibers go through your system relatively intact (think raisins, broccoli, and wheat bran), which adds bulk and prevents constipation. In my opinion, it's not particularly important to sweat the difference because both are beneficial. Remember, the benefit of adding whole, plant-based fare to your diet is that you automatically give your body what it needs in the right form. Mother Nature might even become a friend as you discover Her basic common sense.

In addition to plant foods, consider adding a probiotic to your daily fare. Probiotics are healthy bacteria that assist in digestion, elimination, and immunity. If you are feeling adventurous, you could add unpasteurized fermented foods and yogurt. These are natural probiotics and are even better than the supplements. Also, make sure to incorporate plenty of water into your daily intake. Weight Watchers recommends keeping track by filling a 32-ounce bottle twice a day or a 64-ounce bottle once a day. If you feel that you don't have time for all the peeing, think of it as a meditation break, an excuse to sit down and take a few breaths. Because people often mistake thirst for hunger, drinking more water can aid you in your quest to establish a clearer perception of when your body actually is in need of food. As an aside, I have been told that it is better to drink your water in 16-ounce servings rather than sipping all day long. Your kidneys need a rest too, after all.

The second reason to eat more fruits and vegetables has to do with the nutrients these foods supply. I am sure that you are familiar with the term **antioxidants.** You may not, however, really understand what they are or how they work in your body. In a nutshell (and yes, nuts have them too), your body is constantly exposed to things like pollution, chemicals, and other substances in the environment and in your food, all of which take a toll on your body. Actually, normal metabolic processes, and even exercise, create stress within your body. This stress, which causes mild damage in your body, is called **oxidative stress.** This is similar to what happens when iron rusts or when a cut-up banana turns brown. It is caused by free radicals, which are atoms that possess a charge due to having an excess or deficiency of electrons. These charged atoms scavenge your cells to pick up or deposit an electron, causing oxidative stress, or more literally, creating mild damage to your cells (like rust or a brown banana). Antioxidants neutralize the damage caused by oxidation. They are like applying lemon juice to your fruit salad! Antioxidants appear to bind the free radicals that are created via the normal functions of living, neutralizing them and helping your body metabolize and release them through the kidneys. Antioxidants are vitamins, minerals, and enzymes (proteins involved in metabolism) that are found in whole foods and a variety of spices. Substances (you may notice that I did not use the word "foods") like white flour, sugar, corn chips, soda pop, and hydrogenated oils do not contain antioxidants and are likely to cause further oxidative stress in your body. Think of it this way, when you eat fruits and vegetables (and other whole foods), you are helping your body out enormously as it struggles to survive and thrive in this taxing world.

The third reason to eat copious amounts of vegetables is to maintain proper **acid/alkaline balance** in your body. Now, you may be asking, what in the world does that have to do with my body or with vegetables? Most of us are familiar with the term "pH balance," perhaps in relation to shampoo or swimming pools. You may not, however, have heard the term used in relation to the fluids in your body. This is because mainstream science has not yet established its clear relevance to the body's health and functioning. Doctors are trained to diagnose severe pH imbalances, which are very rare, but they usually overlook low-grade imbalances. Naturopathic doctors are more likely to emphasize the importance of maintaining an optimal pH in your bodily fluids and see it as a vital constituent in your overall health.

A refresher to your eighth-grade science class: pH stands for "the potential of hydrogen." The concentration of hydrogen in a fluid determines its pH measured on a scale of 0 to 14. The higher the number, the more alkaline the solution is. A neutral pH is 7. Levels between 7.34 and 7.45 are optimal in your body. Your body strives to maintain a pH in this range and will pull minerals from your bones and tissues to compensate for acidity in your body. How does the body become overly acidic? A direct cause is dietary.

Some foods are acid-forming while others are alkalizing. Although all foods are exposed to acid in your stomach, the ash (like the ash left over from wood) is different depending on the foods you eat. What foods create an acid ash? If you guessed the staples of our Standard American Diet (SAD), then you would be right. Meat, sugar, flour, alcohol, milk, eggs, coffee, artificial sweeteners, salt, etc., are all acid forming. Healthful foods like yogurt, nuts, beans, and whole wheat are also acid forming. You do not need to eschew all such foods, but the point is to balance them with lots of vegetables. It always comes back to that, doesn't it? Fruits and vegetables are alkalizing. Very alkalizing foods are coconut water, dates, raisins, and spinach. Interestingly, citrus fruits like lemons and grapefruits, which are acidic, actually have an alkalizing effect in the body. So a refreshing, tasty way to begin to alkalize your body is to add a spritz of lemon to your water.

Let's look at some of the possible health effects of low-grade metabolic acidosis (which refers to a chronically acidic system). Think of a day in the life of your body. Lots of work to be done—blood to pump, oxygen to disperse, food to digest, viruses to ward off…And you thought that **you** were busy! One of the many tasks your body is doing is striving to maintain optimal pH levels in your blood and tissues. So how does your body do this if the majority of what you consume are acid-forming foods? Well, your body compensates for this by pulling minerals from your bones and tissues in order to maintain safe pH levels. The kidneys play a major role in this process by excreting the broken-down muscle and bone minerals. Kidney stones are formed when the bones release calcium to buffer acidity and the calcium separates and forms a kidney stone. You can also see how the risk of osteoporosis is raised if calcium is being leached from your bones to buffer acidity. You might consider the irony of eating copious amounts of dairy to fight osteoporosis, when the dairy is acid forming and therefore promotes this leaching of calcium from the bones. Alternative health literature suggests that other potential ills that might be linked to chronic, low-grade acidosis are diabetes, thyroid problems, and high blood pressure.

What you can do: The good news is that this problem is amenable to intervention. You can limit your intake of high-sodium processed foods, increase your vegetable intake, and stay hydrated, possibly adding lemon to your water. Avoid or limit diet soda, alcohol, and coffee. Try to replace some of the meats and starches you consume with fruits and vegetables. If you are curious and want to measure your body's pH, you can pick up some testing strips at your local health-food store in order to get an average of your body's pH. This test is done with either urine or saliva. (These recommendations come courtesy of Dr. Mark Stengler's *Natural Healing,* Vol. 4, No. 9, Sept. 2008.)

So, hopefully you are a convert from SAD to, well, GLAD, Gobbling Lettuce, Arugula, and Dates (that's my acronym by the way). As you acclimate yourself to this new/"old" (more like our ancestors) way of eating, you will discover that nature has some wonderful things to offer. Your body mirrors nature's intelligence. Fuel your body with the stuff that you are made of. And strive to make your meals delicious. Experiment with different spices and cooking techniques. This will open up a whole new culinary world for you that will satisfy your body in a way that feels right because it is aligned with nature.

Not Too Much

I am feeling your anxiety rise now. Anyone out there who has struggled with weight likely has visions of paltry portions of bland foods that barely make a dent in the appetite. You can only endure this for so long. The feeling of deprivation is anathema for all of us. It is an aversion that is wired deep into our primitive brains. The idea here is learning to meet your requirements for pleasure and satiety in a way that is also healthful for your body. It is vital that you do not become so deprived that your primitive brain kicks in and threatens a mutiny.

So what does "not too much" mean and how do you incorporate this without triggering your inner starving (angry?) animal self, who might just go ahead and eat down the house? Here are a few thoughts. Know thyself. If you know that you have a habit of, say, not eating much all day and then losing it at the dinner table, you need to coax yourself to eat smaller, more frequent meals or snacks through the day. If you eat protein-rich snacks, you may find that you are less ravenous in the evening. Vegetables can also serve as a great way to tide yourself over between meals. The main trick here (and quite a trick it is) is to examine your patterns with food and discern what habits set you up for overeating. A common pitfall is allowing yourself to become overstressed and overly hungry without planning for your meals. Then you find yourself starving, and stressed, without any healthy food conveniently available. This is when the pizza or fast food present as convenient alternatives that make it extremely easy to overeat without even realizing it. Believe it or not, half (if not more) of the reason you are eating is to calm the stress rather than to satisfy actual physical hunger.

The need to feel satisfied physically is vitally important in our daily lives. Here are a few more tricks for satiety management. When you are "hungry," or "still hungry" after an appropriate meal, try drinking a glass of water or tea sweetened with stevia. Teeccino is a great caffeine-free grain beverage in the tradition of Postum but much nicer in my opinion. It provides a rich after-meal treat with stevia and some nut milk. You may be surprised that you feel satiated afterward. That's partly due to the twenty-minute rule. (It takes your brain about twenty minutes to register satiety after eating). Sometimes it helps to drink a glass of water when you "think" you are hungry, as thirst often masquerades as hunger. Another trick to curb hunger is grabbing a handful of good old carrots (organic if possible). I find them very useful when I want more food that my body doesn't really need or just want a little something to tide me over until dinner. Bearing down on a carrot has a visceral satisfaction, which admittedly is not the same as a bag of potato chips, but does the trick nonetheless. I would also suggest adding a bit of protein or fat to your carrots to mitigate the blood-sugar response. The fat will also help you process the nutrients.

Lisa Delaney addresses portion control in her book *The Secrets of a Former Fat Girl,* which incorporates humor and practical advice as she details shifts in her habits and identity on her journey from heavy to healthy. When eating richer foods, such as oils, nuts, meats, and cheeses, it is important to keep your attention engaged. You may have heard—meat should be a deck of cards, cheese is four dice, nuts are two C batteries, pasta a tennis ball. If you portion things out, it keeps you honest and will help you shift out of your pattern of overeating. If you still feel deprived, I suggest that you fill up on salads and vegetables to compensate. This brings in the healthy foods and hopefully allows you to feel satisfied after the meal. Try to remember that if you leave a little space inside, your body has more room to do the work of digestion. See if you feel better after the lighter meal compared to how you feel after a heavier meal.

Now, I must add a word for those of you who take the "not too much"
tor too far the other way. You, my dear, revel in your ability to push your plate
away, delay your meal just a little longer, and cultivate emptiness as your pleasure. It is so important for you to shift this to compassion for your flesh, feeling into the crannies of your body and the discomforts that you endure. You
can start to tune in to the pleasures of fullness in areas not involving food as
a way to integrate more sensuality into your life and make your body's desires
less threatening. Deep breaths, sensuous oils, smelling fresh flowers, and other
small luxuries of embodiment will help you to eventually give yourself over
to the pleasure of a nice, healthy meal, trusting yourself to stop at "enough."

The "not too much factor" is only a little bit about the mechanics of
your food choices. It is actually far more about your willingness to integrate
attention to your body into your daily life. This is the yoga part of the equation of the yoga of food. I find that most of my clients with food issues
treat their bodies as an inconvenient afterthought that needs to be showered
and presented to the world, but is otherwise ignored. Consequently, stress,
tension, and fatigue build in the body throughout the day leaving you extremely uncomfortable and worn down. The ready pleasure of food can
easily become a trigger to "just let it all go," leaving you quite miserable in
its wake. The "not too much" factor requires that you begin thinking about
your body on a consistent basis, which includes planning what to feed "it,"
and how to soothe and care for "it" through the day. And, actually, you
begin transforming this "it-ness" into tolerance, then acceptance, and finally
appreciation for the vital body that houses your Being. Think of the yoga
of food as letting your patterns with food and hunger be steppingstones
toward developing a more loving relationship with your physical body.

So, let's move on to this more subtle, embodied aspect of the "not too
much" part of the equation. This is really getting into the yoga of food because
it asks you to be embodied and to notice how you feel when you are eating.
You may have heard the advice to eat until you are 80 percent full. This is obviously a subjective assessment. "80 percent full? What the…?" Unfortunately,

there is no meter available that you can hook up to your innards to measure this: "Ding, ding, ding...time to stop." I used to joke with a like-minded friend in college that it was too bad that you couldn't have the equivalent of an orgasm when you had had enough food. "Quiver, quake—ahhhhh—I'm done!" Alas, the 80 percent rule is far more subtle. It requires some deeper engagement with your body, and when our everyday mind is captivated by external things, it is not much help with this. That said, the ability to attune to this aspect of satiety is a skill you can develop through practice and patience. Remember that it takes some time for your brain to register that you are full. I am sure that you have had the experience of enjoying a wonderful, mindless feed and a half hour later feeling wretchedly full. Especially when you are habituated to overeating, it can feel normal to eat to a point of extreme fullness. This is not a good idea, and not only because it is uncomfortable. From a purely physical standpoint, the excess food creates strain in your system, and when repeated frequently over many years, this strain will take a toll on your body. The reason that you feel uncomfortable when you are too full is that your body is trying to send you a message. The good news is that by developing a new habit (the 80 something % full habit), you give your body room to fix any damages that may have been done.

When you are habituated to undereating, you are hyper-attuned to feeling full and stop when you notice any expansion in your belly. Habitually undereating is also problematic because you live in continuous state of deprivation. My suggestion for both sides of the equation is for you to cultivate pauses in your meal, where you stop, breathe and recalibrate. "How am I now?" Then ask the question posed earlier by my client: "Is this good for me?"

Now, I have a rather radical suggestion to make at this point in the discussion. You may discover through this process that you don't particularly enjoy eating. I remember years ago watching a friend of mine eating a banana with peanut butter. It looked quite delicious, though she confided in me at the time that she wished that she didn't have to bother with eating at all and would prefer to just take a pill that would satisfy her needs so she could be done with the whole messy process. I've also heard people exclaim (and have felt this myself) during mindful eating exercises, "Who has time for all that chewing?"

Eating food is a grand claim to embodiment. It entails giving yourself permission to take up space and to receive. Making a conscious, deliberate choice to do this proclaims the fact that you are worth it. Yes, you are worth it! So I ask you to reflect now on whether you feel this way. Are you really worth it? Are you worth the time, attention, and expense of eating good, healthy food? When you don't think so, you find yourself snarfing unhealthy substitutes in desperation due to the inability to claim your right to a healthy, whole embodied existence. The yoga of food asks you to take this step and to claim the right of embodiment.

Homework for Developing Positive Eating Habits

1. Choose a few small, positive changes you would like to make in your eating habits. A negative goal is something like "cut out sweets," while a positive goal is "increase one portion of fruit and one portion of vegetable a day" or "cook one meal a week." It is vital that you don't overwhelm yourself with changes that feel unnatural or forced because you will rebel. Give yourself at least two weeks with one change before adding another.

2. Here is a list of positive changes that are helpful for people who are attempting to shift from SAD to GLAD.

   • Increase fruits and vegetables by one serving over several weeks until reaching the recommended nine servings. Remember to give yourself at least two weeks with each addition.

   • Cook one home-cooked dish a week. Over time, increase your repertoire. It might inspire you to buy a healthful cookbook and begin exploring the world of beans and grains. Try quinoa, chickpeas, lentils, and other earthy foods. Decide when you will do your cooking, when you will shop for the foods, and how you will handle your resistance ("I don't have time!").

• Increase water intake to around 64 ounces a day. I recommend replacing soda gradually with water or tea. Soda, especially diet, does you no favors. It is plush with chemistry that has an unknown effect on your body and it is acidifying to boot. I recommend that you drink water in large portions (8 to 16 ounces at a time) rather than sipping throughout the day. Your kidneys work hard—give them a rest!

• Add a cup of green tea with lemon to your daily intake (lemon increases absorption of antioxidants in the tea).

• Replace white bread and pasta with the whole-grain variety. Over time, you will come to prefer it. Really.

• Commit to sitting down while you eat your meals. That means no car eating or refrigerator-door eating.

• Take five deep breaths before eating your meals. Check in with your tension levels—what do you discover?

• Replace your bottled salad dressing with a homemade one made with a wholesome oil (olive, grapeseed, sesame, etc.), garlic, and spices and an acid such as balsamic or cider vinegar or lemon.

• Check out your neighborhood farmers' market.

• Shift to organics on the "dirty dozen" (in terms of pesticide residue). The list is always changing, but usually includes celery, peppers, and soft fruits such as nectarines, peaches, strawberries, and cherries.

- Roast some root vegetables such as turnips, parsnips, or beets. This is not hard. Peel, wash, chop, drizzle with oil (olive, grapeseed, sesame), put in the oven and bake for 20 minutes or so at 375 degrees F.

- Try replacing two meat meals a week with some non-meat proteins. Sauteed tempeh is good and is a less processed choice than tofu, lentils have a high protein profile, beans and rice are a favorite and can be quite delicious if done with a good salsa, a little avocado, and/or some diced onion.

- Increase your omega-3s with some fish. Canned wild salmon is a low-mercury, high omega-3 fish. Just rinse it off to get rid of the can residue and salt. Other low-mercury choices are small fishes such as anchovies or sardines. Avoid too much tuna, especially the white albacore variety. Tuna is a large fish and consequently chock-full of mercury.

The Karma of Movement

Karma is a concept referring to our ability to intentionally apply causes that bring about desired effects. This allows us to take a more empowered role in the creation of our lives and ourselves. Empowerment and choice are vital components of a healing process. Our culture promises relief from all discomfort if we just get the right shampoo, or car, or bag of chips. Our airwaves are teeming with substances, accoutrements, dressings, and doings that will relieve us of all discomfort. Consequently, we have learned to abhor discomfort. We deem it positively unnatural and some of us make it a full-time job of avoiding it. And the more we try to avoid it, the more it nips at our heels. Yoga teaches us to create "right pain," consciously walking into discomfort so as to, as Iyengar suggests, become experts regarding our habitual response when things become, as they inevitably do, ("Oh, no!") uncomfortable.

Iyengar tells us, "Willpower is concrete, not ethereal." As I have mentioned, he slaps a man's thigh and says, "Willpower is here." Willpower is embodied and not in our minds at all. Grim determination is in your mind and is sorry fuel for the long haul of a meaningful change process. Grim determination is rife with criticism, judgment, and inappropriate expectations. You must learn to tap into a more vital source of energy in order to sustain a change process. The source that I suggest is your body, which you learn to turn on through movement. It is only through active engagement of your body and your heart that you will expand your limits and your endurance.

Let us consider this reconfigured idea of willpower in relation to food. Most commonly, willpower is thought of in terms of your ability to say "No" at the table. "Oh, you have so much willpower," you are told when you pass on the cake. You are thought to demonstrate willpower through your restraint. Iyengar's definition of willpower is very different because it is based upon an active doing rather than passive restraint. Willpower, in this line of thinking, is a forging through, confronting your limits while remaining firm in your intent. This is empowerment in action. How different this is to saying "No" to a piece of cake! Willpower is about actively making yourself larger and more powerful—quite different from defining willpower in terms of holding yourself back. ("No cake, thank you.") However, your everyday mind is a woefully inadequate tool in this practice and enhancement of willpower. It is very easy to succumb to the more familiar, rigid, and deprived place that is ruled by "No." Most of us have a deep abhorrence of this because it is based on avoidance and restraint and will eventually, if not immediately, rebel. The yoga of food helps you to access willpower by turning on your body in a way that enhances and develops your physical strength and personal power.

I'd like you to pause for a moment and reflect on a time that you faced a difficult challenge. Perhaps you made a speech in front of a group of people. You may have been very nervous and considered finding a way to get out of it, but you ended up facing up to the challenge with a good outcome. In this example, you said yes to something that was difficult, you allowed yourself to be uncomfortable, and you followed through with your intentions nonetheless. Afterward, you feel good, stronger, and proud of yourself for the accomplishment. This is an example of willpower in the way I am using the term. You use your will, or intention, to power through a difficult challenge. When it comes to making healthier food choices, I am asking you to reconfigure your idea of willpower in a similar way. Rather than succumbing to a shame-based, deprivation model where you sorrowfully pass on the nachos, pizza, and beer, envying your compatriots who can "get away with it," you instead use your will/intention to empower choices that enhance the health of your body. You are saying "Yes!" to health-enhancing vital foods. You are saying "Yes!" to feeling better in your body. You are saying "Yes!" enhancing trust in your ability to follow through on your intentions. And because your body is such an accessible tool, you can tap into its power at any time to enhance your experience of willpower. When your mind slips into "Woe is me. I'm so fat. Why can't I have some chips?" you can turn on your willpower through your body. This is where yoga and physical movement become the companion, and eventually the motor, behind your efforts to change.

Yoga invites you to notice and become more informed about your habitual response to bumping up against limits. The ability to acknowledge and breathe into, rather than tighten against, discomfort can be cultivated. Consequently, the physical aspect of yoga is an extraordinary help in your efforts to change your eating habits and to become a stronger person. What you will find through your yoga practice is that you are stronger than you think. (Remember, sometimes what needs changing is your habituated thoughts about yourself. If you don't try something because you think you can't do it, you prove your original negative premise. It's a vicious cycle.) You will also learn that, lo and behold, strength develops over time. This knowledge is only developed through lived experience and the yoga mat, which, as opposed to a diet, is a far more dynamic way to discover this vital fact of our lives. I remember someone giving me advice once about dieting. "You know," she told me, "when I have to spend time doing something I don't enjoy, if I'm on a diet, I think, 'Well, at least I'm losing weight.'" I took this to heart as a young girl and would sit passively, reveling in my "ability" to lose weight. I would think to myself, "All I need to do is sit around, not eat, and kill some time losing weight." Not a very empowered mind-set! Doing something that builds your power, rather than sitting around becoming smaller, is a far healthier (and more interesting!) path to wellness.

Iyengar suggests that you "Learn to find comfort even in discomfort." At first blush, this may sound masochistic, or at the very least, counterintuitive to the point of absurdity. But let us hear him out. "To detect diabetes, one takes a test to see how well sugar is tolerated in the body. Similarly the practices of yoga show us how much pain the body can bear and how much affliction the mind can tolerate. Since pain is inevitable, asana is a laboratory in which we discover how to tolerate the pain that cannot be avoided and how to transform the pain that can." This statement flies in the face of our cultural abhorrence of discomfort, yet I must agree with Iyengar's somewhat stark sentiments. Discomfort in life is inevitable. The sooner we accept this and stop trying to avoid it, the better. The practice of yoga strengthens your capacity to bear up to life. Consciously creating and walking into discomfort reinforces your willingness to be uncomfortable and builds upon your capacity to cope. This strength is a reservoir that you can call upon at the dinner table, or the vacuous times between meals when you feel sucked up by your "hunger." You realize that your intentions are stronger than your transient sensations and that uncomfortable feelings, like the discomfort of holding a pose, ebb and flow in an arc that more often than not opens up into something different. You experience the reality that you are larger and stronger than the fluctuations in your body every time you practice yoga. You grow in your capacity to bear up to your own impulses, and eventually to life.

A yoga teacher at my neighborhood studio commented right before the back bend series that back bends get easier as you go. I realized on number four or so that she was right. I also began to notice this same principle when I was running or cycling. My beginning steps are often laborious and weighted.

Once I get started, it gets much easier, gathering momentum and confidence as I persevere. What an interesting phenomenon. The more you do, the more you can do. That's positive karma in action! When I am holding a long back bend, such as bridge pose, my initial reaction is often a fear-based retraction, "I can't do this." Learning to set aside this predictable seizure of my mind is now second nature. The effort becomes burning in my legs, opening through my core, beating in my heart, and I have entered the experience. Sometimes I hate the experience and I notice myself hating it. I am known to make rather animal-like noises as I release the energy of pressing up against the limits of my body and mind. My husband sometimes calls into the room, "That doesn't sound very yoga-like." Or my daughter will query through the closed door, "Mom! What are you doing in there?" When it is over, I am spent by the effort, and I am left with a flush of competence wrought from what my body can do regardless of the limitations of my mind. How I eat now is often in service of providing my body with the best source of sustenance in order to enable me continue to both study and challenge the limits of my fearful mind. This is willpower in action. Notice it is not a practice of restraint, but rather, a practice of expansion and exploration.

Reflections and Goals for Movement

1. What is your relationship to physical movement? What kind of physical activities do you enjoy? How often do you exercise?

2. Explore your relationship to physical discomfort. How do you respond to physical exertion? For some people, especially those with trauma backgrounds, physical exertion can bring up feelings of shame, inadequacy, panic, and even rage.

3. Are you willing to add consistent physical exercise into your daily regime? What kind of exercise/movement is most appealing to you—solitary exercises like running or walking, or group activities like team sports or a spin class? How

much time are you willing/able to commit on a daily basis
(or five or six days a week)?

4. What are your preconceptions about yoga? Some people
have an idealization of yoga, thinking that practicing it will
somehow bring them to a higher plane, while others see it
as weird and esoteric. If you find it attractive, how would
you like to incorporate a class or a practice into your weekly
schedule? You may substitute this for your exercise, though
unless you are practicing power yoga, it is important to have
some aerobic activity in your repertoire.

5. Make out a schedule of your exercise/yoga commitment,
including what you will do, when, and for how long. If you
are new to regular exercise, start out very slowly, say with ten
minutes of a gentle, nonthreatening activity (such as walking
or dancing) twice a day. I am recommending short, frequent
intervals to help you acclimate to the activity while also
keeping the commitment manageable.

6. If you would like to learn yoga but feel intimidated by a
public class, there are great DVDs and CDs to learn from.
Some gifted teachers include Rodney Yee, Patricia Walden,
and Baron Baptiste. *HeavyWeight Yoga*, by Abby Lentz is
designed specifically for heavier individuals.

Your Core Body Beliefs

Core beliefs are a key principle in cognitive behavioral therapy. According
to the theory, core beliefs are laid down in childhood in the form of mental
schemas about the self, others, and the world. Schemas are organized patterns of thoughts, feelings, and ideas that exist at an unconscious, or at least
preconscious, level. What this means is that we are not aware of our beliefs
systems, rather, they comprise the water we swim in and the air we breathe.

Cognitive therapy aims to make your schemas more explicit (in other words, more conscious), thereby allowing you to modify dysfunctional beliefs. Imagine a fish swimming around in a little murky fishbowl who is suddenly lifted up and able to peer into the bowl— "Well now, that sure is a lot of crap I'm swimming around in!" Cognitive therapy allows you to clean up the waters you swim in, thereby creating a different and more hospitable milieu.

Cognitive behavioral therapy does not explicitly address this, but I believe that we develop a core belief system about our physical body that sets the groundwork for how we relate to and inhabit our body throughout our lives. Particularly when there is abuse or trauma, the self-body relationship becomes distorted and creates the foundation for the perpetuation of abuse and negativity toward our own body. The real tragedy is that we don't even know that we are relating to ourselves in a punitive, self-destructive way. Or maybe we know that we are self-destructive ("I shouldn't eat so much, dammit! I'm such a fat pig!"), but we attribute it to our own shortcomings rather than to deep programming that was laid down in childhood when we had no say in the matter.

I had been working with Cindy for over a year. Cindy is a larger woman who is attractive and intelligent—one might describe her as "intense." She looks at me with a strong gaze and can be a challenging client, shifting between being very vulnerable and childlike to more dominant and even verging on arrogant at times. She suffers greatly, not just because of her weight, but from her vacillating moods, chronic self-doubt, and lack of direction in her life. She questions her marriage, being a mother, and berates herself for not having a career. When we are working together, my presence is gentle but firm. I attempt to ground her in the present and help her identify clear, workable goals. "Let's help you embrace what you have created in your life," I'll encourage. "How would you like to enhance your commitment to your health this week?" When she has an "aha!" moment ("Oh, I get it," she'll say softly), her whole demeanor shifts and her face is illuminated with a gentle light of recognition. Her vision clears and she is able to see outside of the narrow confines of her unhappiness and its limited options. At these moments, she is receiving rather than defending, which she was trained to do during childhood. I can feel her taking my words in and not shooting down my suggestions as irrelevant to her needs or the enormity of her unhappiness. Her habitual style of defending is an ingrained habit of warding off potential threats to her well-being. Other people are seen as potentially dangerous rather than nurturing. This defensive stance toward the world is rooted in early experiences of trauma, when basic security has been threatened beyond a child's ability to cope.

Therapy edged around her history of abuse. "I want to talk about 'the abuse,'" she would often say. Bits and pieces came out as the conversation disclosed and then avoided the excruciating details. Her father was harsh and at times very cruel. She witnessed him beat her mother and was herself often the brunt of his violent discipline. She recalls humiliating beatings as a child and at seventeen being chased up the stairs by him and beaten on her leg with a shoe. She wonders if the life-threatening blood clot she developed on that same leg during her pregnancy is related. Her body speaks unspeakable truths. Perhaps even more damaging was being teased about looking like a boy and the veil of shame she donned early in her life due to her weight, her bed-wetting (until the age of fifteen), and lack of peer acceptance. Cindy's grandmother provided solace in her life. Her grandmother's body was large and plush. Her home was quiet and orderly. Cindy would go there after school and there she could have "as much as I wanted." Apple pie, that is. At grandmother's, there were no limits, no humiliations, and the comfort of cookies and baked goods always awaited her. At grandmother's, Cindy was able to let down her guard; however, receiving love came in the form of food, which is how grandmother also soothed herself.

One day in therapy, we were talking about Cindy's weight. She is in her mid-thirties and is well aware that her weight contributes to her health problems, most recently her hysterectomy and the ongoing possibility that her bladder might prolapse. Cindy described her delicious lunch that day—"A

BLT with onion rings. I really didn't eat that many onion rings," she said in a tone of mild defiance. A few minutes later, she announced that she wanted to talk about "the abuse," not food. I told her that we were talking about the abuse. That her method of comforting herself, her "love" of food, reenacted the scenario of pain ("I'm overweight/bad") and comfort ("At least I can eat"). Later in the session, Cindy wept as she questioned if she even wanted to live without the comfort that food provides. Her core beliefs about her worth, and really about life itself, lay right between the lines of her story about food.

The following week, Cindy came in looking a bit lighter than the week before. She began the session in her more impassioned, didactic tone, discussing the evils of the American diet and her new abstinence from coffee and junk food. During this session, we discussed integrating this empowered self with the shamed, hopeless self lurking in the background. "That frightens me," she said. I told her there is nothing to be frightened of, and instead she can embrace this more vulnerable, shamed side of herself with awareness and not abandon her power. She can integrate the firm, somewhat rigid self ("I'm never late," she announced early in her therapy, and she never was) with the chaotic, wetting the bed, bingeing, messy self. This underbelly represents the core beliefs that haunt her and sabotage her deep wish to change.

When I was in my early teens, my best friend was most teenage girls' worst nightmare. At that stage of life, many of us are fully caught up in allowing the physical body to determine our value as a human being. And my best friend happened to be blessed with smooth, tan skin; round, perfect breasts; silky brown hair; and long, slender legs curving into hips that were just enough. I remember being awed by the rhythms of her appetite. Barely a piece of pizza and she was "stuffed." She left French fries on her plate. Mornings I would gleefully finish off her microwave pancakes. Behind my glee was a strong sense of discomfort—"Why can't I be more like her? What's wrong with me?" But my hunger was so strong that I didn't stop to linger in that discomfort for long. Instead it became buried as an accepted fact about me. I was one of those people who ate too much, too fast. I had no idea that this was a malleable fact about me, or that these strong impulses to eat could be held and accepted and worked with in a loving manner. Sadly, my "hunger" became linked to core beliefs that there was something defective, needy, and "too much" about me.

Perhaps you too have always felt inferior in your body, like something is fundamentally wrong inside and the pleasures of the flesh outside of eating are not accessible to you. Or perhaps you consider yourself all too wedded to the pleasures of the flesh, helpless before them. You may feel that the karma of movement does not apply to you. I certainly remember feeling this way. I had dragged my recalcitrant flesh out for a few attempts to run in my early teens and remember feeling that the oft exalted "runner's high" simply did not apply to me. I wrote it off as something that I was excluded from—my body was obviously somehow deficient. "Might as well eat." How I wish I had had a gentle hand at that time to guide me toward more respect and curiosity about my body, though not as "perfect" as others, but with a right to Be nonetheless. It is strange nowadays, some thirty years later, to be looked upon by others as having that coveted thin body, observed from the outside as a smooth economy of intake and expenditure, without the anguish of unmet hungers and cravings. The truth is, and I think this is true for most thin people over the age of twenty-five, that thinness is made up of certain habits that work more of the time than not to balance hunger with satiety. But there is nothing magic about it—it is a door open to anyone willing to do the work. I do not mean thin is available to all, since it is also a product of genetics and body type. But comfort in your body and a sense of ease with the rhythms of appetite, satiety, and exertion can be cultivated by everyone.

When you have food or body issues, you likely feel defined by your weight, as if others judge you based on your body and label you as "fat," rather than seeing you as a whole person. When you feel you are perceived based on your physical body rather than your inner self, it is dehumanizing. Your ego registers this and can easily don the cloak of negative identity given to you by others. Frances Kuffel eloquently describes this experience in her memoir *Passing for Thin.* "I was 'fat.' A noun, not a modification, to my ears it was my definition and destiny. Not remedial but remediless." She goes on to describe a conversation with her father: "'What does—' I paused to spell out the unfamiliar word—o-bee-see—mean, Daddy?' 'Obese,' he grunted. 'That's you.' I knew exactly what he meant. The word tocked across my head like a cuckoo clock. 'That's you. That's you. That's you.'"

For you, there may not be such a defining moment. However, solidifying your self-image around your body as it is seen by others is a common experience for people with weight issues. When your self is defined in this one-dimensional way, you exist as a body that is unacceptable. This negative identity then influences your behavior, which serves to reinforce the negative identity. Again Frances Kuffel chronicles this experience. "A few motivations for eating—safety, satisfaction—prompted half a lifetime's compulsive eating, which in turn made me a fat girl/woman to the world and a whore to food in my heart."

When you struggle with weight, you struggle with core beliefs about your physical competence. While you may be highly competent in many areas of your life, your negative body schema is lived out in daily defeats experienced in relation to food. "I have no willpower" is a conviction that is made true with every sigh of resignation and deferral of a healthy choice. This core belief can be challenged and changed when it is made conscious. When you are able to enter your body and turn on its vitality, you become capable of much, much more than you think you can do. Your body is a miraculous instrument and that is literally right under your nose. When you dare to enter the world of the flesh, you become aware that you are so much more than the apologetic image staring back in the mirror.

This is where some degree of faith is necessary. Remember, we are like snowflakes, all of us are sharing a similar structure and similar capacities that differ only in their unique articulation. You must have the humility and the courage to relinquish your convictions about what is and is not possible for you and throw yourself on the mercy of your flesh. According to Iyengar, "you can always do a little bit more than you think you can." It is here, in the space of reaching beyond what you think you can do, that strength and competence grow. And with every limit that is challenged, more becomes possible after that. Your body can become the canvas, the tangible actualization of your courage to push beyond your beliefs about what you can or can't do, what is or is not possible for you. The trick to this, however, is not to make your faith conditional, based upon external results. And, given your humanness, this is quite a trick indeed. Because we all want proof. Our faith is tepid, timid, waiting for a sign that we are right, or at least on the right track. Learning how to go through the motions in the present, with vacillating degrees of faith, acting as if... This is the space of change.

Reflections on Your Core Body Beliefs

1. Reflect upon your core beliefs about your body. What words come to mind when you sweep your body with your mind's eye? Give yourself a few minutes with this exercise to allow a relaxation of your consciousness.

2. Did you have a defining moment in childhood that solidified a negative identity in relation to your body? What happened and how did this affect you? How do you perpetuate this identity in your daily habits?

3. What are some ways that you can modify your behavior so as to shift away from the reinforcement of your negative belief system? Some examples may include experimenting eating foods you "hate," like broccoli, or incorporating daily exercise into your routine even if you "hate" to exercise.

Non-Violence Toward Your Flesh (Ahimsa)

Ahimsa is a yogic principle discussed at length in many texts on yoga. It is one of the yamas, which are the ethical principles guiding a yogic lifestyle. Ahimsa refers to non-violence in speech and action toward others, and for our purposes, toward your body as well.

Due to our cultural obsession with weight and "thinnitude" (to borrow a term coined by Frances Kuffel), we often overlook the sheer violence that marks our efforts to shape our bodies into acceptability. Kaiser conducted a study among its patients, largely middle-class people with health insurance, and determined 66 percent suffered maltreatment as children, and noted a clear correlation between childhood adversity and chronic health problems later in life (*Psychotherapy Networker*, Sept./Oct., 2010). We learn to treat ourselves as we were treated. The tragic story behind our nation's declining health is that many of us are reenacting tales of despair and dysfunction precipitated in childhood. It is in childhood that you learn a basic attitude toward yourself. If the attitude is one of love and affirmation, you are truly blessed. If it is one of frustration, invalidation, and inappropriate expectations, you have lots of company. The work of healing is learning how to reshape your attitude toward yourself, starting with your attitude toward the very flesh you inhabit.

The first step in embracing the principle of non-violence is to recognize the sheer superficiality with which you likely relate to your flesh. As I have discussed, most of us are so captivated by the appearance of our bodies that we miss out on the miraculous world that lies just beneath our skin. Blood, bone, and vibration. Who thinks about this vibrant, pulsating, synchronized world unless blood work comes back wrong or something hurts? And then the gaze is one of disappointment, frustration, or fear, rather than the appreciation and awe your physical self deserves. There is a long-suffering nature to your body, a willingness to endure many insults, often without a peep, until it becomes just too much. Or maybe your body is peeping, even squawking, but it is too scary to look beneath the skin, or there is too much else in your life that you think you have to do.

Practicing ahimsa toward your body is a commitment to reshaping your patterns of self-care, and even more importantly, reassessing your basic attitude toward your flesh. What is your basic attitude? For many of us, it is judgment, judgment, judgment. The shift in perspective required for a change process to begin is to see the external condition of your body as merely the result or manifestation of what is unseen beneath the skin. The yogic perspective brings you inside yourself and has nothing to do with your looks. So, rather than berating yourself for being "fat," or for not exercising enough, which manifests an attitude of violence, you decide to rehabilitate something that is glorious, albeit in need of work. In Iyengar's words, "You have to create love and affection for your body, for what it can do for you."

The pervasive message we receive in our culture is that we are all in need of "fixing." This is the byproduct of our consumer-driven society. We are products in need of improvement. There is a simplicity in this focus—it pares down the enormity of your work as a human being to something seemingly manageable as you bear down on your own flesh. It gives you a sense of control and purpose in the face of the darkness. However, when you fixate so much on the concrete—your body, the appearance of things—you are cut off from the mystery. This starves a vital part of yourself—your need for meaning and connection—and makes you more vulnerable to turning to food, the concrete, for comfort. "It's as if you were in a spaceship going to the moon, and you looked back at this tiny planet Earth and realized that things were vaster than any mind could conceive and you just couldn't handle it, so you started worrying about what you were going to have for lunch . . . hamburgers or hot dogs. We do this all the time," according to Pema Chödrön in her book *Start Where You Are.*

Food provides a ready focus for us all. For those of us with food/body issues, food is intimately wrapped up with fixing and rehabilitating ourselves, and so stems from self-denigration and negativity. The yoga of food asks you to approach food and your body in a more loving, life-enhancing way. This helps you move beyond your deeply human tendency to fixate, to worry about what's for lunch in order to gain ground in the vastness of the universe.

The Practice of Loving Kindness (Mitri)

May I be filled with loving kindness
May I be peaceful and at ease
May I be well
May I be happy

Mitri is a Buddhist practice that cultivates warmth toward all Beings. Although this is not a concept from Classical Yoga theory, I include it here because it highlights the capacity to love as a quality that can be cultivated within yourself. In the West, it is often recommended that you begin this practice by starting with yourself. Many teachers, including Pema Chödrön, have commented upon the pervasiveness of self-hatred in the West. I have heard that the concept of self-hatred had to be explained to the Dalai Lama because he had never heard of it before and had no frame of reference. Self-hatred is the inevitable byproduct of the culture of narcissism in which we all have been reared. We learn from day one how special and wonderful we are. Or conversely, and perhaps more pervasively, we do not learn this at all and instead are subjected to glorified views of others through the media whom we idealize and envy. At the root of it all are inappropriate expectations about life, about ourselves, and an overvaluation of self that breeds profound isolation.

Mitri means "loving kindness." Nurturing this attitude toward yourself is a radical act and is a precursor toward developing compassion for others. It is antithetical to how we are shaped in this culture. Loving kindness connotes an abiding respect for, and acceptance of, your own experience, no matter what it is. So if you are "hungry" five minutes after dinner, you hold the feeling with curiosity and warmth, rather than the frustration and self-denigration with which you might normally greet such unwelcome stirrings from below. This is not easy work. It requires a radical shift in perspective. Judgment against yourself, bearing down internally, these are habitual patterns that are pre-reflective. Meaning, you don't even know that you're judging yourself, clenching your teeth, or gripping your abdomen. Bringing these patterns into consciousness is the first step toward change. But, and this is an important *but*, just because you are hungry five minutes after dinner and you are holding this feeling with more warmth and acceptance does not mean that you automatically have to react to the feeling by eating. As Pema Chödrön reminds us, mitri is not just about being "sweet" to yourself, or put differently, it is not self-indulgence. Mitri is an attitude that opens up space. We so often react automatically and in so doing we close off internal space. When you feel anxious and "hungry" in the evening and have a bowl of ice cream, you close off space by filling it up with *stuff.* Mitri helps you to cultivate a lighter, more curious attitude toward yourself, allowing you to dare to sit in empty space a little while longer. Learning to identify your internal patterns of judgment, or violence, takes practice. Who hasn't felt the quake of a nameless emptiness after dinner and before bed, the stretch of evening fading into the darkness that has no end in sight? The nights you are able to hold the emptiness in awareness without immediate reaction are small victories that help you to feel a little stronger in the face of life's uncertainty. And the evenings that you don't show such fortitude? These are the times to lighten up internally and notice the judgment hovering at the corner of consciousness ready to pounce.

Janice, in particular, has been shocked by the amount of abuse she heaps upon herself. "I say things to myself that I would NEVER say to a friend." "Like what?" I urge, curious for more detail and also wanting Janice to make explicit with me what is a largely private, toxic habit. "Oh, I don't know. If I make a mistake, I'll berate myself. I'll call myself fat or criticize my body." Janice is trying very hard to stop this. In fact, during sessions she will often stop herself mid-sentence when she catches herself making a self-denigrating comment. Janice is certainly not unique in this habit.

Kimberly, who is a determined member of a twelve-step program, told me matter-of-factly that she once tried to eat herself to death. "What do you mean?" I queried. In a straightforward manner she explained to me that after being turned down for gastric bypass surgery, due to not being heavy enough, she grimly attempted to gain weight. Her efforts culminated one evening in a rage-driven assault from the inside on her hated stomach, which she intended to stuff to the point of explosion. Death by food. Thankfully, it didn't work and when I met her several months later she was firmly entrenched in her twelve-step program and the day-by-day task of taking responsibility for her *stuff.* She still hates her belly with a passion, often quivering with distaste when we talk about it. But at least she is not acting it out on a daily basis with food. As with Janice, when you make your self-hatred more conscious, you are empowered to change your behavior and intercept your habitual thoughts. You are on your way to creating a more affirmative, eventually loving, relationship with yourself.

Reflections on Ahimsa and Mitri

1. How much violence do you perpetuate toward your body? This may consist of actual self-injury in the form of cutting, or less conscious self-injury in the form of unhelpful eating and exercise habits. It may also be more at the level of thoughts, such as incessant criticism toward yourself.

2. Subtle forms of violence consist of chronic tension and negativity, signifying a habit of closing down your internal experience. If you have a compulsive eating problem, you are stuffing internal space with stuff (material things). This points to difficulty experiencing your internal world. Do a body scan from head to toe looking for pockets of tension. What do you notice?

3. In psychoanalytic theory, depression is envisaged as "anger turned inward," or violence toward the self. If you suffer from depression, consider how this idea may be relevant to your mood problems.

4. Unconditional positive regard for yourself is the practice of curiosity and compassion for your own experience. As explained above, this is not about self-indulgence, rather, it is a willingness to be open to and affirm your feelings no matter what they are. How might this practice be of help to you in healing your relationship with food and your body?

5. What are some concrete commitments that you are willing to make in the development of loving kindness toward yourself? Some ideas are creating a self-gratitude practice (remembering what is good about you), or nurturing activities such as walks in nature, hot baths, or regular massages.

Chapter Four

Your Energetic Body (Pranamaya Kosa)

Imagine that you are at a takeout restaurant grabbing a quick bite to eat after going to a doctor's appointment. You are contemplating the menu and assessing what you want to eat, distracted by the many choices and aware that you don't have much time before you need to be back at work. Normally you don't leave the office, so you forgot to tell your boyfriend that you had the appointment. You could have met him for lunch since your doctor's office is quite near where he works. After placing your order, you glance around the restaurant and see your boyfriend. Pleasure floods your body, your heart quickens, and you feel a rush of energy rise up through your core. You wave to catch his attention, eager to see him and connect. Your legs feel lighter and you are about to walk over to him when you notice that he is dining with an attractive woman several years younger than the both of you. They are looking at one another intensely. Shock grips your body. The warmth in your chest turns cold and your stomach clenches into a tight knot that feels like a pit. Your breath stops. You are suddenly paralyzed, unable to move.

Emotions are strong energetic currents that manifest in your thoughts and behavior. The feeling of being angry, having a panic attack, being in love, or as in the case above, being threatened romantically are felt as strong waves of energy in the body. These energetic states are intensely real and dramatic, though unless you express them to others, they are usually invisible. The second sheath of your Being is this energetic body. Emanating through and around your skin, bone, and organs is a buzzing universe of energy. Energy is a real thing in your body—your heart is a pump that is fueled by energy and your neurons exchange information through energetic impulses. Your moods, tension states, and feelings of relaxation are all governed by energy. Yoga brings new awareness to this omnipresent yet invisible aspect of your Being. Through this awareness, you can learn to manage and direct your energetic states with more consciousness and intention.

One of the greatest gifts of a yoga and meditation practice is that it opens you up to an appreciation of the subtle flow of energy in your body. In our culture, most of us are so entranced by big energy (TV, bright lights, loud music, gossip...) that we have lost our ability to attend to, much less marvel, at, the small miracles of everyday life. Many of us, in search of BIG sensation, unwittingly settle for "BIG food." One of my clients recognized that she found excitement in a day based on what she would eat. I don't think she is unusual. David Kessler's book *The End of Overeating* discusses the use of big, chemically enhanced fat and flavor that manipulate our taste buds and brain/stomach chemistry in order to encourage addiction to these substances. These artificially enhanced foods alter, might I even say pervert, our tastes so that subtle, natural flavors are lost on us. Instead, we seek hit-you-over-the-head textures and flavors that excite, rather than satiate, our appetites. Our gastrointestinal tracts have become amusement parks, leading us to seek out the thrills of a roller coaster (think about your blood sugar!) on a plate, or in a takeout bag, as the case may be.

Yoga and meditation are subtle practices. We do these practices so that we can turn inward and settle our attention and begin to notice things like our habitual energy patterns. This journey is a process that takes time and commitment. At first it may feel unnatural, like a waste of time. You may be so used to being continually stimulated that you feel lost when the noise is turned down. Be patient with yourself and with the practices. There is no other way to tune in to the subtle than to go through a period of withdrawal from the normal bombardment of noise. After a period of time, you will notice the feeling of a deep, satisfying breath, the pleasure of releasing a tight muscle, letting go of your jaw, and the gift of attuning to the gentle hum of life right under your skin.

Pitfalls: Barriers to Change

We will now use the traditional yogic concept of prana/energy to shed light on issues that are relevant to a Western lifestyle. First we address several "pitfalls" using the concept of energy to allow a different perspective. The pitfall of resistance is our first topic. Resistance is a powerful deterrent to change, but it can be managed when you have awareness of its energetic pull toward the status quo. We move on to address the pitfall of chronic tension, the pitfall of difficult moods and impulsive behavior, the use of food to self-medicate, and how these behaviors coalesce to create a problematic identity, which has its own energetic current. We then address the pitfall of hunger and how this almighty force can bring you to your knees if you are not well versed in energy-management skills. Then we move into the solutions offered by yoga. First we discuss how physical movement, particularly yoga, is a magnificent tool to address problematic energy patterns. Bringing more awareness to the energetic feel of your body gives you the power to shift out of tense or chaotic energy states without turning to habitual, unhealthy behaviors like overeating. The role that breath awareness has in helping you to relate more consciously to your energy is then discussed. Finally, the role of self-discipline and mindful management of your energy is addressed in relation to how yoga can help you integrate more awareness and conscious management of energy into your daily life.

What You Resist Persists

I first met Brenda about six years ago. She has large eyes whose stare evokes that of a deer in the headlights. She is tall, very pretty, and very thin. She had struggled with food restriction for many years before consulting with me. When she first came in she was very shaken, as in literally shaken, due to suffering a grand mal seizure as a result of electrolyte imbalance caused by food restriction. Brenda can go days without eating and she likes it. "It's like a high, like you can do something no one else can do. I look at the other mothers in the park and the ones who are thin, and I say to myself, 'I know what you're doing! I know what you're up to!'" Brenda had a rather wild look in her eye when she related this to me, and I could literally feel the pull of her anorexia as she spoke. Her weight was stable at the time, however, and she stopped therapy and I didn't see her for several years. Then she came back. She had started restricting again, had had another seizure, and was scared. "I'm done with it this time," she declared. "It's so not worth it." We worked together until she got pregnant with her second child and then she stopped coming again. I heard from her a few years later after another grand mal seizure nearly killed her. Thankfully, a friend was with her and called the paramedics, who were able to save her life. This time I think she has been scared straight. She is also more open to exploring the severe abuse that shadowed her upbringing in a rigidly religious home. She was beaten by her God-fearing father in measured, brutally self-righteous blows with the paddle that hung over the dinner table. Her mother, who also restricts food, subtly resented and undermined her adolescent daughter's growing beauty and burgeoning sexuality. "I can beat you at this game" (being thin), Brenda remembered feeling toward the mother who wouldn't protect her.

If anyone exemplifies the power of resistance, the drift back to the status quo, it is Brenda. Helping her come to terms with the unspeakable issues beneath the surface of her symptoms has been very important in her healing. But look what it took to get her there! And I am afraid that this is not unique to Brenda. Especially when you enjoy the payoff of your symptom, say the high from not eating or the comatose daze from bingeing, it is very hard indeed to give it up. Resistance is held in place by the obstacles to clear seeing identified in yoga as the kleshas. *Attraction:* "Oh, it feels good," like when you bite into that first piece of pepperoni pizza dripping with cheese. Or conversely when you turn down the pizza and revel in the empty pit in your belly, feeling all-powerful for a moment. Then there is *Aversion:* "I will not tolerate that!" Like when you are feeling exhausted and hungry and the thought of another carrot makes you want to hurl— and stop off at Taco Bell. Or, if you restrict food, the thought of feeling full after a meal fills you with unspeakable dread. *Ego* steps in and supports attraction and aversion, announcing, "This is just how I do things, thank you very much." This could also sound like, "I can't do yoga because I'm not flexible." Or "I don't need to eat like other people do." And of course there is *Fear,* who says, "God, no, I can't handle that!" This strong feeling might be called up by fearing others will see you as incompetent if you can't keep up in a yoga class. Or fear of living without your habitual comforts, "What else is there?" But most of all, we fear what lurks behind the symptom—the untold abuses, shames, and regrets that many of us harbor just beneath what is visible. The only way to loosen these knots formed by the kleshas is by facing the fears and feeling into the aversions. This means identifying what you are avoiding and accepting its presence in your life. If you dread the starkness of life without the comfort of food, you must feel into this by stepping away from the habitual use of food to fill space. You face your aversion to loneliness, which opens a new possibility. You have reached behind your symptoms and done something different and that is outside of your habitual pattern. A pithy slogan from Overeaters Anonymous tells us, "If you want to find out why you're eating, stop eating." And of course, for Brenda, it is the inverse, "If you want to find out why you're not eating, start eating." We must go to that uncomfortable place beyond our habitual pattern in order to feel into what we are avoiding. Yes, you will resist the change, but you can harness the power of your intention, feel the resistance, and make a change in spite of it.

Familiarize Yourself with Your Pattern of Resistance

I know that I am not alone in resisting my yoga and meditation practice. I was tickled one day when an excellent yoga teacher at my neighborhood studio announced during the beginning sequence, "Everyone in here is resisting, including me." This made my own pattern of resistance more conscious for me, as well as transforming it into a shared experience. I have learned that it is not particularly helpful to ask "Why?" or even "What?" you are resisting. Instead, just feel it, make it conscious, and get interested in the energy of your resistance. For me it is an inner contraction, a pulling away that is best phrased as, "But I don't wanna!" or "I'm scared." Of what? Of whatever. Of being too tired, feeling too much, showing up, being seen, engaging. I have learned that the "I don't wannas" and the fear dependably recede and often transfigure into a "Bring it on!" mode toward the end of a practice. The arc of this cycle has become familiar and predictable for me and is applicable to other endeavors in my life, including writing this. It is the great secret of action, and we all know this on some level. You know that once you start something it's really not so bad. This includes your taxes, cleaning your closet, and your yoga practice.

Your resistance will show itself in various ways, such as:

"I don't have the time."
"I'm not very good at it."
"It's boring."
"I don't have the time."
"I don't wanna."
"My favorite TV show is on."

"I've had a bad day."

"I don't have the time."

"I'm giving myself a break today."

Yoga and meditation provide an opportunity to get to know your patterns of resistance and self-sabotage. If in the past you have taken on a new venture with enthusiasm and vigor only to have it peter out within a few days or weeks, consider this an opportunity to re-experience this pattern with more awareness and a different outcome. We tend to repeat patterns throughout our lives (remember samskaras?). As you become more familiar with your pattern of resistance, you become better equipped to ignore it—to wink and smile as you notice your self-sabotaging, defeatist kvetching and carry on with your larger intentions for yourself regardless.

It is important to get really familiar with the pattern and energy of your resistance. Visualize your retraction of self, the inward pull of your body into self-protection mode. For me, the "I don't wannas" mentioned above are coupled with a physical experience of withholding energy right before I go into the yoga room. It is hard to describe, but I feel it as a wash of fatigue coupled with a dollop of fear and a sprinkle of doubt. If I had to visualize myself, I would be collapsing inward in order to protect my energy. As an interesting aside, when it's an afternoon yoga class, I notice that my ankles are often a bit swollen before class and then less so afterward. So my resistance is both physical and emotional. By getting to know this pattern, it need not be threatening or "bad," but rather a matter of fact. With awareness, you can counter your resistance by gently coaxing yourself toward the unknown. And over time, the unknown becomes more familiar, and you remind yourself that you know that you will feel better after you practice. It becomes known terrain that you trust yourself to navigate.

Anticipate Resistance

The next step to managing your resistance in a more conscious way is to anticipate it. I want you to think about the repetitive excuses listed above as a news ticker monotonously circling around your experience. Resistance is ubiquitous. It is also boring—it offers no new information and seeks to keep the status quo. It's no big deal if you learn to recognize it, label it, and carry on with your commitments in spite of it. The more you do this, the easier it becomes and your resistance becomes weaker relative to your intentions. This gives you a feeling of great strength because you develop the confidence borne of knowing that You, your intentions, your values, and your capacity for change are larger than your resistance. Each repetition offers you the opportunity to do something different, but you have to be ready for the magnetic pull back to the status quo and determined to hold to the road of your larger intentions. As Iyengar says: "Humans innately resist change because we feel safe with what is familiar and fear the insecurity that comes with something new. We tend to live in a familiar fixed routine and try to avoid accepting or even feeling what is beyond the known... We seek freedom but cling to bondage."

In the process of committing to a yoga and meditation practice, you can expect to bump up against a lot of resistance. For one thing, although sexy yoga pants abound in magazines and shops, the spirit of the practice of yoga and meditation are not supported in our cultural milieu. The spirit of these practices has very little to do with, in fact is antithetical to, a fixation upon how you look or image enhancement. Furthermore, in our daily lives most of us are inundated by to-do lists and are juggling various demands in what can feel like a nonstop race to the finish line. Because "everyone else is doing it," it lends this style of living a veil of normalcy and even virtue. Although you may know that this is a very dysfunctional way to live, running from commitment to commitment, collapsing in front of the TV at night, grabbing takeout food on the way home... it feels "normal" because this is what you are used to. You also may feel as though you have no choice given the various demands on your time. You have to trust that by giving yourself over to the unfamiliar, new vistas of experience and possibility await you.

Here's how anticipating resistance can help. Let's say you promised yourself that you were going to go to yoga class after work three evenings a week. It is Wednesday evening and you are preparing to leave work after a stressful day. You feel like crap. You have a pile of undone tasks on your desk and your habitual pattern would be to grab a snack and plow through it. But you made that commitment to yourself, "Damn…!" You also remember your last conversation with your therapist and how you both agreed that you needed to be prepared to face your pattern of flaking out on your intentions. That settles it. Tired of the years of broken promises to yourself regarding exercise and remembering how good you felt after class on Saturday, you schlump out of the office and head to the studio. You get there just in time, dreading the practice because you are so tired. What if you can't keep up? The thought of a cool glass of wine and the news sounds so good. The young girl at the desk checks you in and greets you with a big smile. You warm in response. The class starts out in child's pose and the teacher holds the room in silence for a few minutes, merely suggesting that you connect with your breath. You feel very safe in the shared stillness. The weight of your body sinks in to the mat as your arms stretch over your head. You are surprised to feel your eyes well up a bit as you connect with the amount of tension you are holding in your body. You lift into downward facing dog and feel the blood flow through your aching shoulders and into your head. You have entered the practice. A new pattern is being born.

Allow a New Perspective

Remember the pictures you may have seen in school as a child where if you look at it one way it appears to be a vase, but then if you look at it with a different focus you see the profile of an old woman? This is a great example of how our perspective can get captured by one way of doing things, or looking at things, when another possibility is right there, "hidden in plain sight." When you change your perspective on a "problem," often you see that the problem actually hides a gift. Perhaps the pain created by your relationship to food has allowed you to be open to this book and will help you to re-prioritize your commitment to make more room for self-nurture in your life. In order to begin seeing the "problem" differently, however, you must first clear some space that allows you to have a different perspective on your life. Essentially, this means that in order to see the problem differently, you must DO something different. A shift in perspective only occurs when you break out of the familiar pattern/samskara. As long as you are doing the same old thing, you will see the problem in the same old way. In the example above, if you had plowed through your work and then gone home and had takeout food in front of the television, you would have conceived of the problem in the same old way. "I have no willpower." "I always self-sabotage." "I'm just too busy." But because you did something different, you see the problem differently. "I carry so much tension in my body." "I have been so driven in my life that I haven't learned to take care of myself." This new perspective comes from a place of empathy and self-love, rather than from a self-punitive and defeated place.

Reflections on Your Resistance

1. Look over the list of excuses for non-action (or continuation of self-sabotaging behavior) and check off the ones that you most commonly use.

2. Reflect further on your pattern of self-sabotage. How often do you make internal commitments to take better care of yourself? How long do you usually stay with these commitments? What reasons do you give for foreclosing on the process? (Remember, foreclosure means aborting your commitment when it gets difficult rather than holding form in the face of discomfort.) I am guessing you might

be surprised to discover that your pattern of foreclosure is relatively consistent. This is actually good news because it allows you to see the stagnant quality to your resistance and can spark curiosity about what lies on the other side.

3. Now make a list of your intentions for the week. How often do you plan to meditate or do yoga? When will you practice? How will you manage your resistance?

The Energy of Chronic Tension

I recently saw a new dentist. He came highly recommended by my hygienist after my old dentist ran away to Hawaii. I had had a lot of faith in my old dentist and assumed he was keeping me in the know about the state of my oral hygiene. Apparently not. My new dentist is a very affable, young-looking man who means business. "Yep," he commented to no one in particular as he examined my mouth, "this one's an A-plus grinder." "I am?" I inquired, genuinely surprised. "I'm not just a clencher?" "Nope," he said definitively, "you are an expert, long-term grinder." He went on to explain the mechanics of the situation in my mouth and the dire results of this unconscious habit. "My god," I thought to myself, "imagine if I didn't do yoga!" After this appointment, I became acutely aware of my clenching. I noticed the grim set to my jaw as I rushed through various activities, the fear nipping at my heels that I wouldn't get such and such done in time. The pressure I continually put on myself to finish this, that, and the other thing before taking off to accomplish one more must-do on the list. It's taken a toll.

Many people, like me, unwittingly walk around in a state of internal tension. This creates a mood that can quite easily plummet into depression or spike into anxiety. The tension is unconscious and is perpetuated by unhealthful forms of self-soothing, like overeating or overdrinking, which create a drugged state of exhaustion and numbness that masquerades as relaxation. Relating this to yoga terminology, chronic tension is a samskara/

habit that is lodged in your energetic and physical body. Because it is all you know, you are not consciously aware of it. Like me, someone has to point it out to you. The tension is perpetuated by your thoughts and labeled with words like "stressed," "pissed," or "overwhelmed." The tension is primarily physical and energetic. What I mean by this is it is not caused your thoughts or your urgent to-do list. These are just the hooks that you hang your internal tension on. The tension is lodged in the physical tissue and energetic feel of your body and in order to begin addressing it, you have to enter the world of your physical/energetic body.

Yoga provides a platform for you to begin noticing your chronic tension. You are in class standing in Warrior I, which is a strong standing pose often performed near the beginning of class to warm the body. You are aware of the burning in your legs and then the teacher says, "Relax your jaw." "Oh," you think to yourself as you soften the back of your throat and jaw, "I didn't realize I was holding my jaw." As you soften your physical body, you notice a shift in the feel of your whole body. This is an energetic shift that was precipitated by releasing your jaw and goes on to create a cascade of changes in the energetic current through your body.

I was leaving a yoga class the other day and started chatting with the woman sitting on the couch. "Sorry," I said, as I clumsily grabbed my bag and accidentally jostled her, "I'm in a yoga zone." "Isn't is amazing?" she replied, "you just never leave a yoga class feeling bad." I concurred wholeheartedly. "You are so right," I had to elaborate, "sometimes after a run or the gym I just feel drained, but not after a yoga class." This is the energetic magic of the practice. The way the teacher starts out by coaxing breath into your body. The conscious movement that is synchronized with your breath and shifts rigid or jangled patterns in your body into more rhythmic states. As you repeat this practice, a new awareness is borne in your mind-body that you can take off your mat. You begin to notice your holding patterns away from the mat and you experience the magic of how awareness automatically brings a change to your internal state. You can also go through the motions of a downward dog or forward bend on your own and benefit from the shifts these humble movements automatically create in your energetic body, particularly the more you practice them. As my teeth grinding habit so clearly shows, these patterns go deep and developing awareness is a process, coming in layers as you are ready for them. This illustrates the need for patience with yourself as you travel along the path.

Reflections on Your Tension Levels

1. How much tension do you carry from day to day? Some ways to assess this are your level of worry, your ability to allow things to not be perfect, and your ability to sleep and enjoy yourself.

2. Where do you store tension in your body? Common locations are the jaw, shoulders, and the stomach.

3. What are some positive ways that you could begin addressing your tension more proactively? Some examples are starting a yoga or meditation practice, taking a real lunch hour (as opposed to a "working lunch"), or taking a walk in the evening.

Food and Your Mood

Many people use food as a means of self-soothing. This can range from a reward after a hard day, comfort in the face of disappointment, or a salve for a chronically tense body and mind. This might sound like, "I'm feeling depressed, what can I eat?" But often the use of food for mood management is preconscious and habitual, meaning you don't even realize food is a crutch because it's such an ingrained habit. This applies to individuals who use food indiscriminately, without even pausing to reflect on hunger levels or mood states. A big bowl of ice cream in front of the TV is just what you do. The underbelly of this kind of habitual self-soothing is that although it serves as a form of self-medication for depression, anxiety, or stress, ultimately it only reinforces the problems. We will address this habit from an energetic perspective, conceptualizing food as a form of energy you use to shift problematic energy states in your body.

The unconscious use of food to self-soothe was an ingrained habit for Wanda, a forty-something woman I had been working with for years to address various issues. Compulsive eating was just one on a list including severe anxiety and marital problems. When I first met Wanda, she was a member of Weight Watchers, and had even trained to be a leader. At that time, therapy focused on helping her manage her chronic anxiety, which had spiked after her husband got drunk one night and informed her that he no longer wanted to be married. Devastated by the fear of abandonment, she clung desperately to the hope that she could fix the marriage. Her husband went along for the ride, dutifully attending couples counseling and going through the motions of marital life. Wanda's anxiety worsened. She began gaining weight, angrily eating the brownies he insisted on making with her daughter without regard for her issues with food and compulsive eating. Finally, after discovering that he was involved in an affair, Wanda's anxiety grew to a point where she could barely function. She shook all over, could not eat, and had trouble containing her tears in front of her eleven-year-old daughter. Over the next year, she made tremendous progress, finally accepting the fact that the marriage was over and finding a full-time job as a physical therapist after several years of not working. She continued to struggle with her weight and her eating, and it served as an anchor through the brutal period of dealing with her husband's behavior and negotiating the divorce. During this trying time, she gave herself leeway to eat what she wanted and comfort herself with food. After she was through the divorce, she wanted to move forward and part of this, in her mind, involved shedding the extra weight she had gained.

Change was very difficult for Wanda because her evening pattern of compulsive eating was so driven and habitual that she was hard-pressed to identify the triggers to her overeating. Rather, she described "just finding" herself in the kitchen eating, usually without even having an internal conflict of "I want to/I shouldn't." The habit had become more ingrained over the past stressful year and seemed to function on its own accord, sweeping her along in its tide. Even before the year of her divorce, Wanda had had a long-standing pattern of using food for comfort. As a skinny kid, she could eat whatever she wanted. Adults would wag their fingers and say, "You'll pay for that later," but never bother to discuss good nutrition or mindful eating habits. Now Wanda was trying to strong-arm herself into losing weight. She would be very concerned about her weight during the day and would often subsist on an Ensure until dinner. Then, in the evening, when she was letting down from the day, she would consume large quantities of junk food while watching her shows on TV. This was her "reward" for the day. Her concerns about her weight, so prominent during the day, were put on the shelf until morning. Then she would awake depressed and anxious, ready to face another day of penance.

This disconnect between cause and effect is not uncommon for people who chronically overeat. This is not due to lack of intelligence! Well, let me rephrase that—this is not due to lack of cleverness. It is due to lack of intelligence, if we define intelligence in the yogic understanding as acting in ways that truly benefit us. Because we live in a very clever society, many of us suffer this form of lack of intelligence. Wanda's disconnect from seeing the connection between cause and effect with regard to her compulsive eating was caused by her urgent need for self-soothing. Wanda's long day of stress and starvation created such a press of internal tension (think "bad energy") that her logical mind (if A, then B) was literally not accessible to her in the evening. Instead, driven by stress, loneliness, and the intense need for soothing, she was hell-bent to make herself feel better the quickest way she knew how. Her habit/samskara of using food for comfort lit up in the evening, and nothing was going to stop her.

A positive step for Wanda was joining Weight Watchers again so that she introduced more conflict into her evening pattern of self-soothing. In her case, introducing conflict into her habitual nighttime eating was good because she needed some motivation to bring awareness to her driven eating pattern. In addition to her eating disorder, Wanda has a virulent anxiety disorder, marked by constantly second-guessing her judgment, her parenting, and her basic acceptability as a person. Charming and engaging at one level, she suffered an ongoing litany of self-doubt just below her smile. Wanda powered through her days by suppressing her fears about her competence and ignoring the internal press of anxiety. Her core fear was that she would be discovered as incompetent and chastised by a punitive authority figure. This is not a pleasant way to live! The "energetic" component to her bingeing reflects her need to bring a "yes"—some permission and relief—into her inner world of self-doubt and negativity. As self-destructive as her evening binges were, they actually represented her attempt to take care of herself and balance her chronic fear with some pleasure and relief. By joining Weight Watchers, she introduced some conflict into her experience of evening bingeing/self-soothing. Taking away this ready salve for tension\ temporarily increased her anxiety. However, by interrupting this samskara/pattern, she opened a path to discover more beneficial habits of self-soothing. She began walking her dog after work, and after a few weeks found this to be a far more satisfying form of stress release. "I never want to walk Buddy when I get home because I'm so tired, but once I get out the door I am so glad that I made the choice. And I notice I'm not as tired when I get back."

One of the first things to give way when facing negative mood states is healthful food and exercise choices, especially for those who do not have positive habits/samskaras around eating and exercise. A negative mood can so easily envelop you, becoming your "reality" and erasing the valiant goals you set for yourself in a more positive mind-set (was it just this morning?). The urgency for soothing in the moment supersedes all other intentions. "I don't care" takes over and initiates a domino effect of negativity in your behavior, like bingeing, which brings on more destructive thoughts and behaviors, like self-hatred, procrastination, and social withdrawal. Physical depletion often contributes to the urgency for sustenance and comfort that accompanies a depressed or anxious mood. As you develop more awareness of your habitual anxiety or depression, you may notice that you use food to soothe the tension of chronic anxiety. Food can easily serve as a "yes" in a world of "no" (i.e., contraction and negativity). Perhaps soft, billowy, sumptuous substances allow a brief relaxation of your inner girdle of tension. Or eating crunchy, salty textures allow you to release the pent-up frustration that you don't allow yourself to express directly. In contrast to the tension of anxiety, depression is a pushing down of energy in your life so that you are chronically depleted. Food can then be used as an energizer, a way to pump yourself up to face the next task, or it can be the reward to get to at the end of a task. If any of these uses of food apply to you, it is important to recognize that you are using food to self-medicate—and NOT beat yourself up for it. This requires you to bring a tone of mitri, or self-love, to your understanding of your pattern. You recognize that your use of food has served a purpose in your life, you have needed its support in the past. At the same time, it is vital that you develop skills to work with your tension, or suppression of energy, in ways that guide you away from using food as an energizer or soother. The yoga of food involves putting food in its rightful place in your life and not relying on it for energy/emotional management.

Reflections on Food and Your Mood

1. Reflect upon your habitual ways of coping with uncomfortable moods. What methods are self-destructive and serve to reinforce your negative feelings? What are your healthier, more productive coping methods?

2. What role does food play in mood regulation throughout your day? Does it provide something to look forward to? Or is it more a source of guilt and stress? Perhaps it is both.

3. What are some ways you can bring mitri/self-love to your problematic moods and intercede when you are vulnerable to overeating? Some ideas are journaling, music, taking a bath, or resting.

The Energies of Mood and Impulse

We all know that feeling of being carried away and doing something that we shouldn't but just not caring at the moment. You are caught in a wave of energy and you are swept along in its current. "So what?" you think to yourself, "I'll deal with the fallout later." Sometimes impulsive behavior comes after a wave of intense energy—say being really angry and then throwing something. But sometimes impulsive behavior sneaks up on you and carries you along in a subtle grip that you barely notice. The yoga of food involves getting wise to how this form of impulsivity can create inadvertent overeating and sometimes more drastic binges.

I cannot tell you how many of my seemingly civilized meals have been tarnished by the inadvertent pattern of impulsivity. For example, let's say I plan to go out to dinner with my husband. I look forward to it during the day, perhaps not eating as much as usual so that I will be sure to enjoy the meal. I tell myself that I am not going to overeat, but don't think about it too much. We arrive at the establishment pleasantly hungry and are seated. The dining room's ambiance is pleasant and sophisticated, the clink of silverware and wineglasses adding to the busy yet serene feel. The waitress introduces herself; she will be "taking care of us" tonight. I relax into the pleasure of being cared for. Then comes the wine and a pleasant buzz. "More wine?" the waitress appears and graciously refills my glass before she takes our order. "Oh, thank you," I murmur, enraptured by the moment. We choose carefully and then sit back and await good things to come. First the savory salad with lightly dressed greens, just the right proportions of crunch, sweet, and creaminess. The bread is crusty and resilient, delicious with a little butter. Our appetites whetted, we are ready for the entrées, glancing up from our conversation when we catch a glimpse of the waitress in our vicinity. "Your entrées will be right up," she assures us, noticing our eager looks in her direction. The entrées arrive and we descend into them. I don't stop to consider how hungry I actually am at this point. The sautéed vegetables are tender and delicately spiced, the meat falls apart pliantly with just the right amount of resistance, the creamy potatoes bind it all together. "How are your meals?" the waitress inquires. "Don't interrupt me," I think as I reply, "Delicious, thank you." "Would you like dessert?" Our waitress appears with the dessert tray after clearing our plates. "I'll have the lemon tart," says my husband. He's a sucker for lemon desserts. "I'll bring two forks," our waitress assures us. At some point during the entrée there was a peep from in my body-mind, "Melissa, you've had enough. You should stop." The food tastes so good and I just don't want to hear it. "I'll deal with it later," comes my habitual response as I give in to the impulse to keep the stream of pleasure coming. Dessert arrives and the rest is history.

Impulsive behavior rarely has positive outcome and often leaves a big mess to clean up. The above scene is a rather minor example of giving in to impulse. Yet for me, the repeated abuses of my digestive system has created fallout that I am still trying to clean up. But at the time, these consequences don't seem to matter. When you are in the grip of an energetic impulse that has a lot of current, it is very difficult to withstand its thrust. When it has built up without your awareness, by the time the wave hits, the force is much greater than your powers of restraint. Although I had a vague awareness of my tendency to overeat, I hadn't actively planned a way to manage it. Thus, I was helpless in its current, especially after a few glasses of wine. Such ignore-ance commonly results in a food binge, an anger attack, or even having unprotected sex. The release feels good in the short term but the results can be dire, even life changing.

Vanessa does not have an eating disorder. She does, however, have a mood disorder wherein she experiences "meltdowns" that render her a "crazy woman" far removed from her usual contained, highly articulate, and insightful persona. Vanessa is in her early forties and had recently left a demanding corporate career when she contacted me. She sought therapy due to periodic episodes of out-of-control behavior, wherein she would act in a highly uncharacteristic way, like drinking large amounts of alcohol and driving away from her boyfriend's home in an inarticulate state of rage and shame that defied translation into words. Helping Vanessa communicate these profoundly distressing states using language and name the precursors to her meltdowns was an initial step in gaining some control over these episodes. This is similar to what I did above when I named the precursors to my overeating and identified my habitual pattern of denial and self-sabotage.

Your ability to understand and name fluctuations in your mood and energy is fundamental to your ability to manage your impulses—in general and around food. You develop an understanding of your patterns, the precursors to impulsive acting out, and the unfortunate outcome of your behavior. The yoga of food helps you begin working with a more long-term view of your behavior in relation to food and to bring impulse control to your choices regardless of what your mood is like at the time. This will look and sound something like this—"I am feeling really depressed right now. I am physically depleted and feel bad about the comment so-and-so made to me. I am feeling like things will never change. I don't care about being healthy because I know it will never happen. I want to eat that piece of cake (that whole cake?) because it's the only comfort I have. But I also know that I need to find a better way to cope when I feel bad. I am going to walk around the block and then see how I feel." Notice that you did not say, "I am not going to eat the cake." Rather, you left it open, but made the huge step of delaying the impulse by interceding with another activity. This takes an ability to distance from the negative feeling, rather than being enveloped by it. This delay helps you develop something called the Witnessing capacity in your consciousness (we call this the observing ego in Western psychology). The Witnessing capacity helps you to distance a bit from the immediacy of your experience and observe your patterns. This can open up space for you to make different choices, as you see that your patterns are not actually "you," but rather behavioral and emotional habits/samskaras.

About seven months into treatment, Vanessa came to a session looking quite distraught. She gave me a look of despair in the waiting room and walked barefoot into my office carrying her sandals, one of which was broken. "This is just a sign of how my day is going," she said, gesturing to her shoe. She listed the litany of things that had gone wrong that day, missing her workout, the computer not working, breaking her shoe… But the real cause of her despair was not her broken shoe or malfunctioning computer. Rather, it was the creeping fear that she was not getting any better. "I went for a walk yesterday and the only thing that I felt was, 'I did it.' I don't feel joy anymore." Her determined attempts to do the right things to feel better (exercise, eat well, and socialize) were seemingly not effective in lifting her mood. "I don't want to live this way!" she sobbed. Her fear of never getting better was the theme of the session. My job was to provide her with the containment and perspective that her parents had been unable to provide when she was a child. I was firm in my stance that she was getting better, that her feelings of despair, though real, were not accurate reflections of reality or her progress over the past several months. I spoke to her about her childhood history (when she was left in her room to tantrum for long periods without parental intervention) and how today she was re-experiencing the abandonment and desperation she had felt as a little girl when her only form of coping was to rage and scream. We discussed how she would take care of herself the rest of the day. She promised not to drink alcohol and agreed to share with her boyfriend that she was having a "bad day." This was hard for her due to her shame about being so "weak" and unable to function normally. If Vanessa had food issues, she likely would have overeaten in response to her despairing mood. The danger for her was overdrinking and then raging at her boyfriend. Our session was well timed because it interrupted the pattern and brought awareness to the usual stream of events so that she was able to manage it differently.

Vanessa came in a few days later looking much more relaxed and calm. She had made it through the other day and agreed with me that things were not as dire as they had seemed. She also agreed that it made a world of difference that she had not acted out and "made a mess," but rather allowed her mood to pass. She had the insight that even though something may not feel very good in the moment, like taking the walk or not buying alcohol, it's like an investment in the future that you collect rewards on at a later time. "I felt really good when I woke up today because I realized that I made it through a really hard time without making things worse." We discussed how the next time she has one of these days, she will have a concrete experience of containing her mood without acting out and making her despair tangible in "bad" behavior, thus reinforcing her feelings of being weak and broken. She now knows from her own experience that although she is suffering in the moment, the feeling will pass and she will emerge whole on the other side. She is on her way to developing mood-management skills that will aid in her quest to find meaning, and eventually joy in her life.

Mood management and impulse control require a larger perspective that allow you to see yourself experiencing a mood, rather than being the mood ("I will always feel this way!"). If you have an understanding of some of your challenging energetic/affective patterns, then you know that no matter how wretched you may feel at a particular moment, the feeling will pass. You also know that you can either make a mess by acting out, for example, by overeating, or you can find an alternative way to cope that keeps the broader perspective of your well-being in mind. You begin to appreciate the arc of your moods, recognizing that they reliably shift and how you cope with them has huge impact on your well-being on the other end of the mood. These observational skills are like muscles in consciousness. If you haven't exercised them much, they will be rusty, and it will feel very unfamiliar. It does get easier over time as you dare to delay destructive behavior and instead learn to witness your emotional tides. Yoga is a tool that will help you build these muscles. It provides skills and guidance to self-soothe and thus, interrupt destructive patterns of behavior with different behaviors and a different attitude.

Reflections on Your Mood and Impulses

1. What negative moods do you frequently suffer from? Some examples are depression, anxiety, pessimism, low motivation, or feelings of futility.

2. Assess your mood-management skills and impulse control. Are you able to contain strong feelings without destructive behavior? Can you contain a strong urge to do something that will have harmful consequences or do you often find yourself surveying the wreckage of your negative behavior?

3. How do the capacities of mood management and impulse control relate to your issues with food? Do you act out difficult affective states with food? Do you have difficulty containing impulses to eat unhealthy food that your body does not need?

The Energy of Identity

Cindy, whom you met in the section on Core Body Beliefs in chapter 3, came from a home with a physically and emotionally abusive father and a passive mother. Her mother was unable/unwilling to protect Cindy from her father's unpredictable outbursts. Then in her late teens, Cindy experienced a significant cycling accident which caused her to be hospitalized and in rehabilitation for several months. These traumatic experiences coalesced to form Cindy's view of the world as an unsafe place where she had little power to protect herself. Learned helplessness is a concept from cognitive behavioral psychology that describes the impact traumatic experiences have on a person's sense of self-efficacy, which is another term from cognitive behavioral psychology, referring to a person's perception of his or her ability to effect change in the world. When you are exposed to traumatic situations in which you are powerless to protect yourself, you learn that you are helpless. Consequently, you do not attempt to improve your plight when conditions change and you can impact a situation. Your "story," meaning the way that you link meaning to the events, is that you are helpless. Your identity supports this story and you unwittingly support a victimized plot line.

During her psychotherapy experience, it became apparent to me that Cindy filtered her experiences through the lens of being a victim. Though "true" in her early life, this framework now resulted in her negating her ability to effect positive change in her life. Cindy has a binge-eating problem. She re-creates the "story" of being a victim by allowing the impulse to eat and the rhythm of the binge to overpower her, again and again, giving up her power of choice and reinforcing the story of her victimization and powerlessness. Her relationship to food and her weight are just one expression of passivity in her life. Things happen to her, rather than being chosen, or co-created, by her. Her marriage, her job, her home, her body all are unsatisfactory things that she feels powerless to change. The energetic quality underneath her storyline of being a victim is a weak, collapsed pattern that she repetitively re-creates in a food binge.

Who you *think* you are carries a distinct energy. It has an energetic hold on you that makes it very easy, in fact at times irresistible, to keep doing the same things over and over. We create and re-create ourselves everyday. And there is an energetic force that keeps us stuck in creating the self that we may want to desperately change. These are our samskaras, or habitual patterns. The yoga of food is so powerful because if you believe that "you are what you eat," then changing what you eat gives you immediate power to begin re-creating who you are. Pretty exciting stuff! However, changing the "stuff" of your body also involves bumping up against the energy of your current identity. The hard part is that you must be very patient with this process because your current identity isn't going to want to let go. In the gap between applying new causes and seeing their effects the energy of your current/old identity will creep in like a slithery snake, "Who do you think you are, eating a salad? Don't you know that this is a losing proposition? You don't ever stick to anything." These thoughts may be conscious, or more likely, they may be felt at an energetic level—a smoke screen of pessimism clouding your actions and veiling your mood.

A term I often use with clients is "collapse." This is an energetic word. Your system collapses beneath the weight of the negative story line you keep telling yourself about yourself and keep making true with your behaviors. When you have a self-system that is dominated by a negative story line ("I am helpless"), it takes a lot of psychic energy for you to function. Consequently, your energy gets worn down by self-doubt and feared judgment from others. You are vulnerable to collapsing into a heap of helplessness when the demands of others and the world become too much for your flagging self-system to support. There can be a bizarre kind of comfort found in just giving in to your despair and reinforcing the energetic force of your negative identity. Having the rage, or the binge, and succumbing to your feelings of inadequacy feels like a relief due to the strain of functioning under the burden of chronic self-doubt. Some people actually find comfort in thoughts of suicide, "I'll just check out and it will be over." Vanessa described feeling cleansed, albeit shamed, after a meltdown and indeed she often showed renewed motivation to change following an episode. This obviously creates a negative pattern/samskara that is deeply damaging to your self. At worst, the pattern of collapse can become an identity that you live out by perpetuating a view of yourself as a damaged person, a perpetual patient/victim who is beyond help. Or periods of better functioning can be punctuated by intermittent collapses that continually bring you back to square one. Learning to connect with both your pain and your power is vital in the healing process. Your collapses are both habit and choice. "I can't" is a toxic story line in your life that you make true every time you collapse. You must learn to affirm your feelings, no matter what they are, and also make a choice to not self-destruct in their wake. Put differently, you learn to tolerate your own energy without acting it out.

Cindy recognized that she wanted people to feel sorry for her. She craved recognition for the suffering she had endured, but in her effort to obtain this, she undermined her own power and self-esteem. I reflected to her that living out the story line of being a victim sabotaged her deeper wishes for health and well-being. Giving up her need for others to feel sorry for her necessitated that she learn to validate her own suffering. By affirming the realness and the difficulty of her past experiences (her story), she can grow beyond her need for others to validate this for her. This is an energetic shift wherein she honors her own experience and feelings, and provides a container for this within her own body, heart, and mind. Cindy must bring value to her interior experience, rather than depend on others to validate her through their recognition.

When you create a container for your experience, you can approach your experience with regard to its prominent story line, or you can slip beneath the story line and instead relate to the energetic quality of your experience. For example, "I am depressed because ... " or "I feel anxious about ... " are typical, story-based ways we relate to our experience. This involves dealing with the particulars of a situation, the content regarding what happened and why you feel so bad. It can be helpful to journal about these aspects of experience or talk about them with a friend or therapist.

Another approach is to not focus on the "because" or "about" (in other words, the story line), but instead get interested in the energetic quality of your mood state. You may notice that whether you are anxious about an upcoming event or ruminating about a difficult relationship, the energetic feel of your anxious mood stays consistent. Likely your throat and chest are tight, your stomach is contracted, or perhaps your shoulders are hunched. Energy tolerance provides a space wherein you learn to acknowledge and make room for your painful feelings on a physical/energetic level. The details of why you are feeling bad are not so important. Providing a container for your moods means that you allow yourself to feel a certain way without acting out your feelings, for example, "I'm depressed, might as well eat." As your tolerance for feeling bad grows, you may come to see that no matter what the particulars of the story line for your low mood are ("I'm lonely." "I'm fat."), the predominant themes such as "I'm a loser," or "nothing ever works out for me," in addition to your physical experience (clenched stomach, tight jaw and shoulders), remain consistent day to day and even year to year. And this is actually not bad news. Rather, it helps you get to know and accept yourself more fully. You know what your core issues are and therefore you are not surprised when they are tweaked. You bring the gentle voice of mitri, loving kindness, to your experience.

Cultivating an *integrated, body-based level of awareness* allows you to disengage from the righteousness or permanence of your feeling state (your "story") and to instead notice the transience of, and variability within, your moods. An integrated, body-based level of awareness means that you integrate what is happening in your body with your conscious mind. You develop an understanding that your moods live in your body, while the story line lives in the ego. The ego seeks to solidify and make "true" your story line, no matter how bad it is. At least it's familiar, the ego says, "At least I know who I am." Your body, on the other hand, holds a more complex and changing reality. Yes, some of the ego's labels and designations are true, perhaps you are feeling anxious or hopeless at the moment. But these conditions are changeable and fluid. Begin to notice the variability of your mood by connecting with the ebb and flow of energy in your body. By not solidifying your mood ("I'm depressed. Always will be. I'm going to bed."), you have an opportunity to act differently. This might sound like, "I'm having one of my low, hopeless days. I'd like to just go to bed, but I think if I take a walk around the neighborhood I might feel a little bit better." You interrupt the habitual pattern by introducing a new possibility. Your body feels a bit different after your walk and now something else is possible. Perhaps you feel able to call the supportive friend who told you to feel free to call when you are having a rough day. Rather than blindly acting out your story line and proving it true with self-sabotaging behavior, you open a new door where that may lead to a different outcome.

Reflections on the Energy of Your Identity

1. Reflect upon your "story" about yourself. What are the primary themes from your childhood? How do you perpetuate this story line in your life now?

2. Can you relate to the concept of "collapse"? How do you negate your power in your daily life?

3. What are some activities that you would be willing to try to intercede when you are headed for a collapse?

But I'm Hungry!

I have had clients tell me that they believe they may have been starved in a previous lifetime. Many a person has lamented, in the safe confines of my office, "But I'm hungry!" The impulse to eat and the experience of hunger is so often laden with frantic need, entitlement, and fear. People who have habituated to our food culture automatically interpret any twinge of discomfort in the body as "hunger." Even the thought of having a salad for lunch may bring of a crashing wave of hunger/deprivation. The kleshas are at work here, particularly *attraction* ("Oh, it's so good!"), *fear* ("I'm scared to be deprived!"), and *ego* ("Don't tell me I can't have it!"). These obstacles to clear seeing become deeply entwined with your eating patterns and cause you to go terribly astray. After many repetitions reinforcing habitual, driven responses to the kleshas, emotion and physiology are working in concert to create strong "hunger." Well-intentioned plans to lose weight or be healthier don't stand a chance when confronted with this powerful drive from within. However, by getting curious about your experience of hunger, you bring more consciousness to your habitual response to it and can begin to gently introduce positive changes.

Iyengar, in his discussion of pranayama in *Light on Life*, suggests a pause after exhalation. However, he warns that if the pause is prolonged, "you will feel a sudden lurch of panic and suck in air more greedily. This is our instinctive attachment to life reasserting itself." I believe that the intensity and ferocity with which many people relate to food is connected to this "lurch of panic," when the instinctive attachment to life is threatened. I have felt it myself when hungry and feeling a threat from within or without that my sustenance may be revoked. This is a primordial, energetic clutching to life, greedily taking in. You may know cognitively that your life is not in jeopardy when you feel strong hunger, however, the primitive energetic state of clutching subsumes your capacity to respond more consciously. This reaction is especially true if you are a serial dieter and have learned to expect deprivation as your due. Waiting too long to inhale is the same thing as waiting too long to eat, or not eating enough, which is the intermittent fate of the serial dieter. If you aren't on a diet now, it's only a matter of time until you will be. Expectations of deprivation have become lodged in your body-mind and will create the lurch of panic, which captures you in its immediacy. Bringing more awareness to your emotional and physical associations to hunger will widen your experience of hunger from this reactive lurch to a more curious and exploratory position.

Hunger is very subjective and it is very fickle. It is physical, it is habitual, and it is emotional. You can begin to relate to your hunger with regard to its energetic feel in your body. You likely know what I am talking about when I use the words and phrases "starving," mildly hungry, "just right," and "stuffed." But do you really know how these states feel in your body? Do you have a sense of how hunger starts in your body, how it shifts from stomach to limbs to chest to mouth? In starting to examine its fluctuations, you begin to take note of its vagaries. Most of us have experienced the sensation of being very hungry and for whatever reason, not being able to eat, and having the hunger go away (or change into emptiness that is not experienced as hunger). Physical hunger, like the emotions, has an arc. It starts as a vague sensation in the body; it grows and peaks, then subsides, then re-emerges, and then subsides again. Hunger is not a static physical state. Becoming more aware of this variability is helpful because it creates a space where you can become more curious about, and less reactive to, your experience of hunger. You realize that it is an energetic pattern that ebbs and flows, grows and recedes. The lurch of panic is not a permanent state. In fact, it is not a helpful place to eat from, since it is reactive and anxiety-based. It is far better when you wait out the lurch and eat from a place of relative calm.

Hunger need not be a problem, at least amongst those of us who are blessed with an abundance of food to eat. It is your associations to hunger and your reactivity to the sensations that create difficulty. If you interpret hunger as a problem, if you feel threatened by it and tense yourself against it, then you will have a very hard time responding sensitively to your body's actual needs. Because your response to hunger is so habitual, it takes practice to slow down and actually tune in to how hunger feels in your body. The second layer to this awareness is getting familiar with how you interpret the sensations of emptiness, gnawing, or fatigue, which accompany hunger. Do you become anxious, preoccupied with quelling these feelings as quickly as possible? Do you live in deprivation mode, as if someone is standing over you ready to snatch your food away? Does your stomach or jaw tense as if you are preparing for battle? These ingrained reactions are your problem—not your hunger. You will meet Sophie, discussed below, who felt a vague shame around the pleasures of eating. This is but one example of the odd associations to food and hunger that are often just beneath conscious awareness.

Geneen Roth has written many books about compulsive eating. She writes sensitively about the need to tune in to the feelings lingering beneath the compulsive eater's obsession with food. She points out the harsh judgments that the compulsive eater has about her body and her needs, as well as the rigidity with which she approaches food, her body, and her needs. Roth's work with women focuses on differentiating between emotional hunger and physical hunger and helping women learn to not respond to the former with food. She advises that physical hunger be approached with kindness and sanity.

Tune in to your hunger, decide what you are hungry for, create a nice place to eat, and enjoy.

Her advice is wonderful in its simplicity and inherent respect for the body wisdom we all share in relation to how to feed ourselves. I fear that for many of us, however, her advice is simply not enough. I do not mean to imply that some of us are inherently flawed or unworkable. But given the physiologically and mentally ingrained samskaras/habitual patterns of people who have been misusing food, in addition to the nutritionally distorted foods we are surrounded by, the world of physical hunger becomes a terribly complicated one to navigate.

For most people hunger is emotional. Pleasure, satisfaction, guilt, anticipation, excitement, disappointment, boredom ... This is but a mere sampling of the conflict-laden responses many of us have to what lies before us on the plate. I've heard that the stress levels endured by waiters and waitresses rival that of air traffic controllers. What does that tell you? Your waitress may not have the lives of others in the palm of her hand as she slings dinner plates to their respective owners, but she might as well have if one were to gauge this by the enormity of others' reaction to a late or botched order. Given the emotional intensity with which so many of us relate to food, it can become extremely complicated to distinguish between emotional hunger and physical hunger. Yes, there are clear-cut situations of binge eating in the absence of any hunger. But, more often than not, binges, and even just ordinary overeating, are triggered by hunger and the emotions surrounding hunger. These emotions, which can range from shame and panic all the way to giddiness and entitlement, can easily hijack your ability to interpret what your body needs and when you should stop. This lays the groundwork for poor food choices, mild overeating, or an actual binge.

Most often there is a gap between hungry and sated. There is a moment, right after finishing a reasonable portion, but before any satiety has registered in your body, that you may feel a strong desire (a "lurch") for more. This quake of hunger is intense and in the moment can feel permanent. I believe it is here, in the gap between not enough and too much, that compulsive eaters and bulimics (and maybe even Joe Schmoe) lose their way and seek to stuff this gap with stuff—with the material. The ability to sit in this space, to recognize its transience, to not be engulfed by it, this is the fruit of getting more familiar with the energies of yearning and impulse. In this gap between "not enough" and "too much," the distinction between physical and emotional hunger becomes an arbitrary one. Rather, the ability to tolerate your own hunger and emptiness, whether physical, emotional or a melding of the two, is the space of healing. Bringing compassionate awareness to these vulnerable energies feels better than any scarfed pizza, burrito, or ice cream sundae.

My husband's maternal grandmother, who has since passed, was in her nineties when I first met her. She was a dignified, elegant older woman who garnered great respect in the family due to her stately bearing, kindness and firmness in just-right proportions. I had to laugh after Christmas Eve dinner several years ago when we were cleaning up and she found a tiny juice glass to save the smidgen of fish stew that was left over from the meal. I looked at her and said with great feeling, "A woman after my own heart!" I too hate to throw away food. Now, I am guessing that her issue stemmed from having lived through the Great Depression, while mine stems from living through my own smaller-scale depressions. It brings up a deep sense of loss for me. My husband gets annoyed with the foods I must put in the freezer to eat another time, knowing that months later the freezer will be overflowing with indistinguishable plastic bags filled with ice-encrusted foodstuffs that are beyond recognition. If you have a similar attachment, I challenge you to experiment with throwing away small quantities of food. This will help you to work with letting go and to feel into the emotional aspect of your hunger. When you are more comfortable with these emotional tides of longing and need, you will be better able to accurately interpret the concomitant physical sensations of hunger.

Hunger amongst the well fed (as opposed to those who literally don't have enough to eat) is primarily an energetic pattern in the body-mind. Its force brings you to your knees and you seek anchoring in the material realm as you grab something to eat. And then you get lost in the lull of the rhythm of feeding—the act of chewing, swallowing, incorporating, it feels so good you don't want it to end. It is so easy to lose touch with the energetic world of feeling, which though subtle, will tell you when you are full. It is also easy, in your dread of becoming lost in "not enough," to cross over into "too much." You anchor yourself in the domain of the concrete, the annamaya kosa/material body, as you seek to fill the gaps of your own emptiness with "stuff." And here, in the ever so concrete realm of "too much" ("Oh, my aching stomach!"), at least you know where you are—you need to eat less. Conversely, for those of you who do not eat enough, the dread of "too much" supersedes the sensations of hunger. The challenge on both ends of the spectrum is similar—learning to integrate the concrete with the energetic and to trust your ability to do so. This means listening to the subtle impulses sent by your body and brain, and then responding to them accordingly. You learn to appreciate the sensations of satisfying hunger and learn to withstand the quake of emptiness that may shudder through you when you have had "enough," knowing that it will pass.

Cultivating the capacity to calm the frantic response you may have to hunger is strongly related to the section on breath below. I urge you to read over the breath meditation a few times when you get to it and really feel it in your body. This gives you a concrete tool to work with as you seek to interrupt an unhealthy, habitual response to your experience of hunger.

Reflections on Your Experience of Hunger

1. Do you find yourself feeling frantic, entitled, compulsive, rigid, or angry around food? Which of the kleshas (unclear seeing, attraction/aversion, ego, fear) are at work here for you?

2. Do you relate to the idea of food as anchoring, a return from the more nebulous energetic body to the material world? How do you feel when this anchor is threatened, e.g., by a diet? What are some ways that you can anchor yourself without

using food? Some suggestions are breathing, walking, or connecting with a friend.

3. Experiment with quieting down and tuning into your breathing before eating. What is it like for you to sit with hunger without immediately eating? How does hunger feel in your body? What emotions come up in response to your hunger?

4. Expand your food journal from what you are eating to focus more on how you feel after you eat certain foods. This is an opportunity to explore their energetic effect on your body. Notice how particular foods affect the quality of your hunger at the next meal.

Yoga-Based Solutions

Your ability to move and transform your own energy is a vital component of your relationship to food. At the most basic level, food is energy. Client after client has told me that food is their "comfort." As mentioned, I think that taking in energy (ingesting food) is a preconscious attempt to shift internal energy. Again, you can think of it as an internal "yes," allowing a softening of painful and constricted energetic states. The yoga of food helps you to use food for what it can do (provide nutrition to your body) and to distinguish that from what it cannot do (soothe an anxious mood or lift you out of depression). This section will ask you to experiment with a new way of managing painful or disorganized energetic states. Rather than medicating moods through the passive taking in of food, I am suggesting that you experiment with moving through "bad energy" using your breath and body. I use the word "experiment" to give you an exploratory attitude in this endeavor. You are not committing yourself to anything—you are just opening to new possibilities.

Creating Energy Through Movement

I remember as a young girl, probably around fourteen and before I had any positive experience with exercise, thinking to myself, "Who would want to exercise? It takes so much time and work. It's really rather messy. Why not just sit around and eat less?" It seemed like a no-brainer. How wrong I was! The point of exercise has little to do with the calorie burn. It has everything to do with the energetic shift it creates in your body-mind. Yoga is a special kind of physical movement that is meant to be done with more mindfulness than ordinary exercise. This aspect of the practice is very important because it lights up consciousness in your whole body. Daniel Siegel, a psychiatrist and researcher on attachment and the brain, defines the brain as the "distributed nervous system" that integrates the whole body. This is a very interesting way of defining the brain because it takes us out of our head and into our bodies. So, although the electrical/chemical connections of our nervous system may be most concentrated in our heads, our "brain" extends down our spine and into our gut and extremities. Many of us live in our heads (preoccupied with cycles of repetitive thoughts) and do not enjoy connection or integration on this bodily level. Yoga engenders more integration through mindful breath and mindful movement. "Mindful" means that you bring consciousness, or attention, into your experience of your body, "Oh yes, my shoulders do feel really tight." Or "I guess I'm really not that hungry after all. My stomach feels like a fist and I am hardly breathing." That said, I believe that mindless exercise has a place in mood management and the yoga of food as well. When you are very upset, a downward dog and deep breathing can be helpful and grounding. So is a brisk walk around the block. The point is, you must begin to cultivate the ability to interrupt a negative energetic state with movement rather than relying on food. In fact, movement is the quickest, most effective way to impact your body-mind, and this will help unhook you from your dependence upon food. When you move, you breathe more deeply, your heartbeats quicken, and you are automatically brought out of your head and into your body. This may not be a pleasant place to be at the moment. However, it beats being disconnected from your body, which begets more destructive, self-sabotaging behavior. Sooner or later, you will have to come back home to your flesh, and the sooner you return, the less painful the reunion will be.

In my own experience, I often resist moving my energy. I am tired, frustrated, or preoccupied and it just seems like too much work. This resistance was especially true for me in the past, when I was experiencing more difficult, virulent energetic states. I learned through the repeated experience of moving through my resistance and doing it anyway (at that time, "it" was running), that moving energy in my body, inviting the expansion of my chest and lungs, increasing the beating of my heart and rhythm of movement in my extremities, flushed the negative energy and helped me shift out of very painful states to more manageable ones where I could direct my energy into fruitful pursuits, like journaling or even just doing the laundry. This experience of shifting my energetic state from a disorganized, sometimes chaotic, state to a more relaxed, coherent state was so powerful that over time physical movement became a primary coping tool for me. This does not mean that I no longer experienced resistance to exercise. I almost always at least slightly resist any activity that requires me to intentionally expend energy. But my resistance pattern is so familiar to me, and I am so used to ignoring it, that it exerts less and less power in my day-to-day life. My yoga practice has been fundamental to learning about and accepting these patterns in my body and has helped me engage more fully in other activities, like running and cycling.

Physical movement provides a tool to recalibrate your energetic system. Through your body, you begin to challenge your mental and emotional habits of resignation, avoidance, and withdrawal. Actions are a much more powerful way to impact your energetic system than attempting to change your thoughts, especially at the early stages of change. Through physical movement, and most particularly through yoga, you tap into the universal power that already exists within your own body. "The material body has a reality that is accessible. It is here and now, and we can do something with it," according to Iyengar. Physical movement is a means toward not feeling at the mercy of your negative energetic patterns. Learning to bring consciousness into the body is a skill and a habit. And it is essential in learning to manage food issues. It is also a way to develop self-efficacy in relation to your own body. Remember, self-efficacy is a term from cognitive psychology that refers to confidence in your ability to initiate and effect change. When you have a food disorder, you lack self-efficacy with food and with your own body. Extremely competent, intelligent individuals dissolve into helplessness before the lure of certain combinations of fat and carbohydrates. According to yoga theory, it really has nothing to do with the actual tempting food and more about the relationship you have with your own longing and impulse. If the energetic states of longing and impulse are suppressed and sequestered, ensconced in shame, they will hijack any ability you have to refrain for a greater good. Think of Wanda's nightly binges after work when she was driven by a toxic cocktail of fatigue, stress, and denied hunger. If, however, your longings for comfort and impulses to indulge are known and tolerated internally, if you know they are merely energy patterns that you can move through, then you know that you will survive their thrust and come out whole on the other side.

I am always tickled when a client discovers the power of physical movement, particularly if it's yoga, under my watch. Miranda consulted me due to chronic depression that had begun about six years ago when she had moved to the area with her new husband. Miranda was twenty-nine when she finally decided to seek help. She had been against therapy because it seemed "weak" and believed that she should be able to get out of her funk on her own. Miranda was able to function adequately enough to get to her job as a bank manager every day, but when she came home in the evening, she was wiped out and ended up watching television and not doing much else. Miranda felt she was overweight, and this was a big source of contention in her marriage. Her husband was an ex-competitive swimmer who worked at a swim shop and coached part time. Miranda was the primary breadwinner, while her husband spent hours in the pool or hanging out with similarly inclined friends. Their marriage was marked by lack of communication, lack of shared time together, and lack of warmth. She was furious with him for his self-centeredness and his rejection of her, yet she did not express this directly to him and really didn't even admit it to herself except on rare occasions when she was overwhelmed by her anger at him. Their marital distress finally culminated with her husband's announcement that he was moving out. Miranda was devastated. However, she was also aware that this was a necessary thing due to the lack of emotional engagement between them. During her therapy sessions, we had at various times discussed her low energy, digestive complaints, and general unhappiness with her body. When the separation occurred, she began going to a local yoga studio that had opened right by her home. She described feeling really good about herself when she would leave the studio after the early morning class and soon she developed a sense of connection with a few of the other students. She told me that it felt very different from her previous experiences working out at the gym: "It's hard to explain," she said. "My body just feels really different when I do yoga. And I had an epiphany the other day in class. I looked around and I realized that I'm not the only one with issues here. I realized that everyone in the room was struggling with something. I found it comforting somehow." Although she was very sad and frightened about her marital situation, she also said she felt stronger. She began looking for another job and was more able to discuss her needs and feelings with her estranged husband. When I last saw her, she was wondering if he was someone who could meet her needs, rather than her former focus on wondering if she could win him back. She was continuing to take better care of herself and exuded a sense of empowerment and confidence that was lacking when we first started to work together.

You must find another way to intervene at the level of the physical body when you are attempting to impact a habit/samskara of the force and depth of a food disorder or, as in Miranda's case, a mood disorder. The good news is that breathing more deeply, pumping your heart, moving your energy, mindfully and mindlessly alike, will help you to work with the energy of this samskara. You lay down new tracks in your nervous system every time you practice these new habits of putting your resistance aside and forging into the unknown world of your body. This empowers you to deal with the realities of your life, which may be very painful, as with Miranda's marital separation, but are far more manageable when faced directly than when avoided and denied.

Reflections on Your Relationship to Movement

1. What is your reaction to the idea that your habit of taking in energy/food to feel good can be transformed into moving energy through your body with physical movement? Do you think this could apply to you?

2. Have you had experiences with shifting your mood through physical movement? How powerful was this for you at the time?

3. What kind of movement are you most comfortable experimenting with when you are in a negative mood state and wanting to comfort yourself with food? Walking is the least threatening activity if your knees and back allow. Yoga, swimming, dancing and cycling are other options. I suggest choosing an activity and beginning to practice it regularly. Then it will be readily accessible to you when your mood hits the skids.

Yoga Practice: Another Way to Nurture

Yoga provides a structure for you to get really familiar with the ebb and flow of your energetic states, including your pattern of resistance and your use of food to energize or self-soothe. Vinyasa yoga refers to a flow of poses that are "placed in a special order." What I enjoy about yoga is that it is very respectful of the energetic patterns that we share as human beings. Yoga sequences usually start out very gently by encouraging deep breathing coordinated with gentle lengthening of the muscles. As the sequence progresses, more energy is built up in the body, allowing deeper engagement of the body, heart, and lungs. The class peaks in more vigorous poses allowing you to sweat, move, and release. You are then brought down into opening poses where you allow yourself to benefit from the flexibility engendered by your vigorous movements. Hip openers and floor stretches are often done at this time. Many people, myself included, find themselves weeping gently at this phase of the practice. You are then guided into savasana, final rest, where you are allowed to let go of everything and enjoy the changed ebb and flow of energy in your body.

The conscious use of breath to warm and energize the body is integral to yoga. When you exercise, you naturally breathe more deeply, though sometimes your breathing can be more like panting, which stimulates the sympathetic branch of the nervous system (otherwise known as "fight or flight"). In contrast, yoga focuses on slow, deep, nasal breathing and brings your awareness to your tendency to hold your breath and "power through" difficulty, a habit that increases stress in your body. When you practice the same sequences over and over, you develop a familiarity with the flow that begins to feel comforting and nurturing. You will find that hanging your head in forward bends and downward dog feels really good at the beginning of class. Some yoga instructors even encourage you to moan audibly as you experience release of tension and increased blood flow in downward dog. As you breathe through your nose, you deepen and equalize your inhalation and exhalation, which has a calming effect on your nervous system. Another soothing posture is lying belly down with your forehead resting on your hands, exerting a slight pressure on your forehead.

You must practice these postures in order to experience their benefits. At first the postures with feel unfamiliar and you will naturally feel awkward or self-critical. You might say, "This doesn't help with anxiety. I feel like crap because I'm so inflexible!" You leave the class feeling demoralized. I implore you to not give up so easily! Remember that we are like snowflakes. The experienced yogini next to you who is communing with her toes in a seated forward bend expresses the potential that lies in your body as well. She has just been practicing it longer than you have. You too can cultivate pleasure and intimacy in your body. Some of the postures are very difficult and you may find yourself full of dread—"Oh god, the back bends are coming." This provides you the opportunity to notice how your tendency to dread things sabotages the moment. Back bends are an opportunity to open the chest and lungs and are thought to be helpful with depression. They are also very challenging because they take a lot of energy. They provide you with an opportunity to gather and focus your energy and stay with discomfort for a few breaths. Over time, you will be surprised at the flood of release that you experience when you come out of the back bend. The poses become like old friends. You meet up with downward dog and your body says, "Oh, yes, I know you. How are you doing today?"

The ebb and flow of discomfort and the rhythm of effort and release is central to what is healing in a yoga class. For me, it has become a metaphor for life. In life, you must engage and then you rest and release. There is a steady rhythm to this (like your heartbeat), and it is good. Yes, a part of me would really enjoy sitting around eating bonbons without a care in the world. But this is not how life on the planet is structured, and I would probably get bored anyway. Learning to accept the flow of life—you work and rest, engage and release, expand and contract—provides structure and safety on a day-to-day, even moment-to-moment, basis. There is a comfort in this flow and you can experience it through your yoga practice. And here is the most essential piece of the puzzle if you have food issues. My conjecture (and my experience) is that food has become your release, your "ahhhhh ..." moment when you let down the pressure and stress for a moment and become a biological creature experiencing pleasure and comfort. We all need this! Especially in our driven society, where so many of us live in a state of exhaustion and fear. However, you must find a way (many ways, really) to light up your pleasure circuitry and to allow a release that does not involve food and does not have a negative backlash. This will take time, practice, and faith. Through repetition, you will create new circuitry in your body-mind. Your old circuitry will still be active, but over time you can create competing behaviors and experiences that will eventually dismantle these old patterns. Yoga offers a nurturing way to rewire your circuitry and to experience the pleasure of release balanced with effort.

Sophie is a rather extraordinary girl who spent her adolescence encased in a ball of flesh. She stopped going to school at fifteen due to the teasing she endured about her weight. Her parents were disengaged, more preoccupied with Sophie's older brother, who had a loud drug problem while she quietly ate. At twenty-two, subsequent to being diagnosed with type 2 diabetes, she lost one hundred pounds in about a year. She achieved this through a combination of rigid determination, small meals exactingly spaced apart, intense exercise, and single-mindedness. She consulted me when she began regaining the weight. "Once I reached my goal, I didn't know what to do. I felt lost so I started eating again." Although it is difficult for her to let go of the rigid schedule of her food and exercise plan, she is learning to trust the rhythms of her appetite and need for movement. After disclosing to me that she went to the gym twice a day for two hours at a time, I asked if she looked forward to or dreaded her workouts. She admitted that they felt heavy and burdensome. She agreed to go to the gym once a day and the following week said that she felt good about this. We are emphasizing the importance of having pleasure in her exercise, as well as with her food. She looks rather sheepish when I ask her what she likes to eat and is surprised when she realizes that she feels a sense of shame when she "admits" to liking peanut butter or yogurt with granola. "It feels like there is something dirty about it." I inquired again if she had ever experienced sexual abuse, and she said she had not. Her body shame stands on its own. We are slowly helping her dismantle this shame, first by making it conscious and next by introducing more pleasure into her daily life. She recently disclosed that she enjoys showers. She is considering starting to swim, as she enjoys the feel of water on her body. She is on her way toward giving herself permission to be in her body and trust the ebb and flow of pleasure and discomfort.

Perhaps some day she will discover yoga practice, but in the meantime, she is discovering the meaning of yoga, union of mind and body, through connecting more sensitively with her body and making more room for pleasure in her day-to-day experience.

Reflections on the Flow of Work and Rest

1. What is your relationship to the flow of work and rest in your life? Dysfunctional relationships to this are evidenced in workaholics or those who "steal" relaxation by procrastinating necessary tasks. Or others who drive themselves to get things "over with" but find that the to-do list never ends.

2. How is your sleep? If you have trouble with sleep, it points to difficulties relaxing/surrendering.

3. Do you use food as an "ahhhh ... " moment of release and nurture? What are some other ways you could allow relaxation and release in your life?

4. As you develop a practice of using physical movement as a coping tool, it is important to bring awareness to how this impacts your breath. Shifting attention inside and cultivating breath and body awareness are vital steps in the healing process.

Energy and Breath

We have covered a lot in this chapter so far—the energy of resistance, the misuse of food for energy management, the energy of mood and impulse, and the energy of identity. Now we are getting into the solutions and addressing breath, which brings us into the heart of yoga. Breath awareness is fundamental to yoga practice and energy management. Breath is the primary way that we nourish ourselves—even more than food! If you are not breathing well, you are not well nourished at a basic level. In this section, we explore this most fundamental way we relate to our bodies at every moment. Bringing more awareness to your breath gives you an invaluable way to energize, nourish, and care for your vital self.

Your breathing is a strong indicator of "how you are." It is impossible to be breathing fully and deeply and to be having a panic attack. It is impossible to be breathing fully and to engage in binge eating. My guess is that individuals who are restricting their eating are also not breathing fully. Rapid, shallow breathing indicates dominance of the sympathetic nervous system and preparation for "fight or flight." Deep, slow, abdominal breathing is indicative of parasympathetic dominance and brings your body into a restorative mode. Breath is a unique function in your body because it is involuntary while also being accessible to your conscious control. This gives you the potential to have enormous influence over "how you are" on a physical, energetic, and emotional level.

Yoga emphasizes a conscious synchronization of breath with movement. Go to any yoga class and the instructor will likely encourage you to breathe through your nose and to gradually deepen and lengthen your breath as class progresses. Ujaiyi breathing is used in vinyasa yoga and is done by slightly constricting your throat (as you do when you whisper), which creates a soft, oceanic sound. Making your breathing more audible is helpful in bringing more consciousness to your breathing pattern. By increasing awareness of your breath, you develop a method for self-soothing that you can bring to your life beyond your yoga mat. For many people, shallow breathing is so habitual that they are unaware that they are breathing in a shallow, constricted manner. By experiencing moments of deeper, fuller breathing during your yoga practice, you have something to compare your habitual pattern of breathing with. "I don't breathe!" a client once exclaimed to me in amazement, after taking some yoga classes. Once you realize how good it feels to breathe deeply, you begin to notice the difference when you are not breathing fully. Bringing more consciousness to your breath through yoga makes it more likely that you will catch yourself breathing shallowly in the car when you are "fighting" traffic on the way to work. You realize that you don't need to "fight" traffic at all as you take some deeper breaths. Cultivating this bodily level of awareness will help you bring more awareness to your food patterns. Taking a deep breath before a binge will likely not do you much good ("the horse is out of the barn," as they say). However, your awareness of your breathing and tension levels throughout the day will make it far less likely that you will be hijacked by a binge at the end of the day.

Pranayama is the branch of yoga devoted to the study and regulation of the breath. If you want to find out more about it, I include some valuable resources at the end of this text. For the purposes of this discussion, I am emphasizing bringing more conscious awareness to your breathing during your yoga practice, and over time, into the rest of your day. This is potentially a life transformative shift. When I do a guided-breath meditation with clients, they invariably tell me that they feel better. Often, I can sense a palpable change in their presence. They sink more deeply into the couch and engage with me in a more real way. Let's try one right now to give you a taste of what I am talking about.

Breath Meditation

Get comfortable in your chair. Begin to feel into your body, shifting your attention from the outside environment to the inside world of your body. Become aware of the rhythm of your breathing. Breathe through your nose and gently constrict the back of your throat, allowing your breath to become slightly audible as an ocean like sound. Notice a gentle expansion as you inhale and a slight contraction as you exhale. This rhythm of contraction and release governs your breath, as well as every cell in your body and all life on the planet. So give yourself over to it right now and synchronize your breath with this rhythm, amplifying it subtly as you inhale and exhale. On your next inhale, gently take in a little more oxygen and as you exhale, extend the release so as to allow a little more room for your next inhale. Imagine yourself bringing in life energy and nourishment as you inhale and imagine yourself releasing tension, waste and toxicity as you exhale. "Inhaling, I take in energy and vitality.

Exhaling, I release all that is not useful to me." Begin to breathe with your whole body, imagining your breath like a gentle wave emanating through you. Feel your chest and rib cage expand more fully as you inhale and enjoy the release as you exhale. Notice the shift in your energy as your breathing slows and deepens. Take a few moments to feel the changes in your body and your breathing so as to highlight this experience. Remember that you have access to this calmer, more relaxed state at all times.

Breathing patterns are habitual and unconscious. Over time, through cultivating breath awareness, you can change your relationship to your breath and use this extraordinary function as a tool to both soothe and energize your body. The benefit, albeit subtle, is also very real. The key here is to remember that you are sitting on a storehouse of untold treasures. You have the key, but you must learn how to use it. Patience, practice, and not a little bit of faith are necessary ingredients to begin enjoying the treasures right under your nose.

Breathing Practices

1. Practice ujaiyi breathing. Start by whispering softly to yourself. Then contract the same area of your throat while breathing through your nose. The oceanic sound is very soothing.

2. Andrew Weil, a leader in alternative medicine, suggests that you conceive of the exhalation as the beginning of your breath cycle and that you follow your breath for a few minutes in this out-in rhythm. Exhalation as a beginning is a paradigm shift for those of us who are overly focused on taking in.

3. Take some deep breaths, focusing on lengthening your exhale relative to your inhale. Try breathing through your mouth when you exhale and push as much air out as you can. This will improve your capacity to take in more oxygen on your inhale. Lengthening your exhale relative to your inhale "turns on" the parasympathetic (restorative) branch of your nervous system.

4. Set your watch or phone to beep hourly. Take three deep ujaiyi breaths, focusing on lengthening your exhale. This simple method is a powerful way to begin retraining your nervous system.

Tapas: Discipline Yourself with Kindness

Tapas is a concept from yoga philosophy that is fundamental to the change process. And no, tapas is not referring to the delicious Spanish tidbits that you enjoy in a restaurant (wouldn't that be nice!). In this context, tapas refers to the heat and gentle pressure applied in order to facilitate a change process. Tapas is wrought from the energy of fire. A common metaphor that is used to describe tapas is putting a soft clay pot into an oven. The heat from the oven creates a reaction in the clay that solidifies it into a more definitive shape and hearty structure. In your own growth process, you generate internal heat through the energy of your determination and you transform this energetic heat of intention into tangible action. It is tapas that gets you to lace on your walking shoes, get out your yoga mat, or go to the grocery store to buy ingredients for a healthy meal. Change occurs when you transform your nascent intentions (thought) into action (behavior). You need not feel completely confident in your intentions, but you carry them into action and the heat generated from this process burns through your insecurity. Through the consistent application of heat, and the ongoing repetition of new actions, pressure is applied to your mind and body, which results in slow and steady change. On a physical level, your body becomes stronger and more flexible. You make more mindful food choices and your body responds with increased vitality. On an emotional/ mental level, you bring tapas to the fluctuations of your feelings and impulses and hold steady in your commitments in spite of the ebb and flow of your emotional state. At first, changes will be subtle. You will notice that you have a little more stamina, a tad more flexibility, or more capacity to hold intense energies in your mind and body without succumbing to the temptation to disengage or explode.

Initiating a change process requires willingness to adhere to some sort of structure (think clay pot) in your daily life. You can begin at the level of the annamaya kosa/physical body and make changes in your daily diet and exercise habits. Though you are at the level of the physical body, you automatically impact your energetic body through your engagement of tapas. You engage tapas when you notice yourself feeling tired or overwhelmed about the changes you are making. This is an opportunity to not repress your feelings, but also not to act on your impulse to give up or self-sabotage. Rather, at these points you can reach for resources that will help you to strengthen your commitment to contend with reality in a more resolute way. These resources can include books, inspirational speakers, or people that you respect and can reach out to for guidance and inspiration.

Janice (of the chocolate syrup episode described in chapter 3) illustrates how people with extreme weight issues often have difficulty employing tapas in their personal lives. Janice is a meticulous employee in a responsible, corporate position. Her home, however, is often a mess and she uses fast food on a daily basis to self-soothe. Though disciplined in her day job, she lets it all go when it comes to care of herself. Janice is split in her capacity to utilize tapas. When it comes to her job, her friends, and her family, she responds to expectations in a steadfast and exacting way. When it comes to herself, particularly her body and her home, she collapses. These extreme polarities are not all that unusual. For many people, it is habitual to be over responsible for others and to neglect the self. Bringing more balance to your life involves pulling back from habitual patterns of self-sacrifice and neglect. This requires tapas on both ends—bringing boundaries to your commitments to others and firmness to commitments to yourself. This is difficult because you risk others' anger at you for no longer selflessly meeting their needs. You have to choose yourself over others, which will feel "selfish" at first. Tapas is needed to sustain healthy commitments to yourself when it would be far easier to do what you've always done and self-soothe in a disengaged, habitual way, for example, by bingeing or watching television.

Janice was in the habit of succumbing to fantasy and consequent dissociating from the realities of her personal life. One day Janice told me that she had gone to one of the Twilight movies. "It was really dangerous for me," she said. She described feeling herself getting pulled into the fantasy the film created. For Janice, this was a trip she could not afford to take because it reinforced a part of her that was already all too active, her capacity to remove herself from the reality of her body and allow her mind to become flaccid and disengaged. Iyengar explains the dangers of this tendency: "When we daydream, we are mixing fantasy and the dullness of sleep... This may be pleasant and soothing, but it leads nowhere. In fact, when we return to present reality, we may find it, by comparison, quite unpalatable. This is a painful state emerging from a painless one."

For those of us who venture too far from the realities of our bodies and our lives, for example perpetuating ill health and stress by dissociated eating, or running up debt on the credit card, we must strengthen our ability to stay grounded in the realm of the real, gradually honing our capacity to contend with reality. This requires tapas, which is firmness in the face of the temptation to fly off into what we wish were the case, rather than contending with what is actually so. Tapas is actually a kindness to yourself, because it will bring about conditions that are far better than the fallout you perpetuate when you succumb to fantasy and denial of reality. The energy of the heat that you generate through your intentions, carried into action, burns through your denial and creates change. Like the clay pot, you, your body, and your life take on a more definitive shape and structure. The energy of tapas effects change in the realm of the real, your body/annamaya kosa. In Janice's case, her ability to recognize her dissociation, and its dangers, was a crucial step in her growth process. This helped her to channel energy into more consistent, disciplined care of her body and her home.

Reflections on Self-Discipline

1. What are your associations to the idea of self-discipline? Do you consider yourself a disciplined person?

2. What are some disciplines that you would like to bring to your daily life?

3. How would you rate your capacity to bear up to reality? Are there particular areas that you are grounded in reality and others where you dissociate? Reflect on the differences between the two areas and why you make this split.

Balancing Your Private Economy of Energy

"I am so tired!" "I am exhausted!" "I'm just so tired, bone tired." Eyes fill with tears as the experience of the body wells to the surface. These sentiments are a common refrain from many of my clients. A daily struggle to press against the limits of the body and accomplish the have-tos on the list. It's heart-rending. My corollary to the term "the worried well" (the folks without severe mental health problems but who are nonetheless unhappy) is *the everyday sick.* We are the people without major health problems like cancer, diabetes, heart disease, or autoimmune issues, but who are nonetheless unhappy in our own skin and burdened by our bodies. Irritable bowel syndrome, thyroid problems, and pre-diabetes are examples of the plethora of problems the "everyday sick" are diagnosed with. Entering the domain of your body/annamaya kosa with an eye to tuning up your energetic system is the focus of this section.

You are an energetic system. As you already know, your energy is a limited resource. You make decisions every day regarding how you spend and how you replenish your precious stores. Energy drains are tasks that deplete you and give you nothing back. Think of negative relationships, obsessing over your weight, and self-abusive behaviors such as bingeing, cutting yourself, or getting drunk. Watching television, although a passive activity, is often an energy drain because it gives little to you and often leaves you feeling lethargic and empty afterward. This is especially true when you watch it in excess. Reciprocal energy relationships apply to things like parenting, work, exercise, reading, and cooking. These activities all take energy, yet they also give energy back in the form of money, love, and increased health and self-esteem. Think of how you feel after spending time with your child in an engaging project where you are working together on something and enjoying one another's company. You might feel exhausted afterward, but you also feel good about yourself and closer to your child. When your life is out of balance, your daily activities take more energy than they give to you, leading to chronic stress. This can set you in a cycle of wearily meeting obligations followed by fruitless attempts to restore yourself through passive activities like excessive TV watching, overeating, or overdrinking. If this is the case in your life, you need to find activities that feed your energetic system in more deliberate and truly nurturing ways. This requires you to become a sleuth regarding your energetic system, taking it upon yourself to assess what activities and attitudes rejuvenate you and what activities and attitudes deplete you and leave you feeling more drained.

The world is full of energy drains—fear, unrealistic expectations, and critical voices circulate around you every day. Likewise, there are many sources of energy in the world. Food, money, sex, music, nature, and other people can all be sources of energy. A healthy individual has a variable and flexible reliance on all of these sources of energy and a fluid relationship between giving and receiving energy. Distortions in energy management are exemplified by people who either hoard energy (for example, eating too much food, attention-seeking behavior, or being miserly) or leak energy (like overspending, talking too much, or engaging in frenzied activity). Many of us fall into extremes of alternatively hoarding and leaking our precious energy. It is quite common to hoard energy in one area and leak in another, for example, overeating food while leaking money. The art of energy management is finding an appropriate balance between what you are taking in and what you are giving out. This requires bringing consciousness to your energetic system and taking responsibility for how you are spending and replenishing your stores.

Individuals with food issues overvalue food as a source of energy. In need of comfort? A reward? Ability to get through the next task? When food is your "go-to" for energetic replenishment, you fall into this category of food overvaluation. Overvaluing food launches you into a negative energy cycle with food. Your energy is often consumed by thinking too much about food and overeating, followed by feeling sluggish and bloated physically and full of regret emotionally. The strain that excess, unhealthy food puts on your body depletes your physiological energy. If you think about it, it is a great irony that the way we are meant to bring sustenance and restoration to our bodies can become a primary source of energetic depletion. Your mental focus on food diminishes the energy you can put into cultivating other, potentially restorative activities. Food has captured your attention and diminished your appreciation of other sources of beauty and enjoyment in your life. I refer to this as "oral capture." Some examples of this are "Yeah, spectacular sunset, love the pinks, but when the hell are we going to eat?" Or "Sure, the sex was pretty good, but dinner, out of this world!" If you recognize this tendency in yourself, be sure not to approach this with a self-punitive attitude. A little humor goes a long way. Think of George Costanza from *Seinfeld*, who in an attempt to bring together his two greatest pleasures in life takes a pastrami sandwich into the bedroom. There he is, in the middle of "the act," emerging from the covers to lustily take a bite of pastrami à la *Nine and a Half Weeks*. So in your own life, just begin to take note of how often you are thinking about food during the day. Note whether you get excessively focused on what you are going to eat for dinner. Do you feel disappointed when you finish a meal? Begin to ask yourself, "What else might be enjoyable, nurturing, or sensual in my day?" You might not come up with anything at first and this is expectable. Asking the question, however, is important and already introduces a new possibility.

The yoga of food asks you to bring more consciousness to your energetic system. I suggest that you bring a wide lens to your exploration of how particular foods, as well as activities and people, feed or deplete your energy. You will discover that all foods and activities have a larger purpose and greater impact than how they feel in the moment. We all know that a bag of chips is pretty tasty and satisfying in the moment. But have you noticed their effect on your energetic system an hour later? Or six hours later? How about the next day? And the six hours of time you burned in front of the TV? How did that leave you feeling the next morning? Now consider the phone call that you enjoyed with your warm, interesting friend from college? The short walk that you took after dinner? The latter two activities are not preferable merely because all health magazines tell you to do them. They are preferable because they impact your energetic system in helpful and predictable ways. Yoga tells us that everything we do has a ripple effect that impacts how we feel and what we feel capable of in the moment and many hours later. This effect is often quite subtle, but when you tune in your awareness, you begin to notice these subtleties.

It is important to consciously take stock of the demands upon your energy and the activities that you engage in to replenish yourself, as well as the ways that you unnecessarily leak energy. Are you like Janice, selflessly jumping through hoops to please others and collapsing in the face of your own self-care? Or are you like Wanda, depleting yourself through a grueling day and then gobbling food in an attempt to regroup? Perhaps you are like me, weeping a river of tears when you must throw away the rotten bananas or wilted greens. Now consider what demands upon your energy are non-negotiable and what energy drains are self-sabotaging behaviors that you can change? What non-oral methods do you have for self-soothing and replenishing? Remember, passive activities like watching TV are not particularly restorative. It is also important to remember the ripple effect when you are making choices about what to eat and how to care for your body. You can get curious about how certain foods affect your energy for the day and even the next day. When choosing foods to eat, you may not only ask, "Is this nutritious?" but also, "How will this affect my energy and physiology?" When you eat, you can think to yourself, "Let this nourish my whole body." You begin to send restorative intentions with the food you eat, which will positively affect your energetic system. This increases your motivation to make intelligent choices, realizing that the choice will go down your throat in a short period of time, but the food, and the intention with which you ate it, will have ripples you will need to contend with for many hours. In the same vein, you may notice, as I have, that if you start the day off with yoga or meditation, you are in a mind frame to make healthier food choices for the day. And when you've eaten well the night before, you are more likely to practice yoga or meditation in the morning. A positive samskara is in motion!

Reflections on Your Personal Economy

1. List all of the demands upon your energy. Include obsessive thoughts and mind games you play with yourself on your list. Then note beside each item if it is a reciprocal relationship (it gives you something back—for example, reading to your child) or an energy drain. Put check marks beside the energy drains that are optional, like negative relationships or rumination.

2. Now go through the list again. Look at the energy drains that are optional. Write down some concrete ways you can change this relationship so that it is not so draining.

3. Reflect on the ways that you hoard energy and the ways that you leak energy. How can you bring more balance to these distortions. Do you need to work on procrastination (that is hoarding energy), budgeting your money, or not gossiping? Do you think that you would have more energy if you shifted these patterns?

4. Assess your methods of energetic restoration. How much do you use food to energize, motivate, or comfort yourself? What are some non-oral options to this that you would like to cultivate?

Savasana

For those of you who have taken a yoga class before, you are familiar with savasana. It is placed at the end of a class and it consists of lying in a prone position where deep relaxation can occur. Its purpose is not only to allow the student to recover after a possibly strenuous practice, but also to allow absorption of the practice before running off to accomplish more tasks. We so often do not absorb what we take in—be it food or other sustenance. We frantically race along, taking in and checking off tasks without assimilation. In the spirit of encouraging more conscious assimilation, I am placing a brief savasana here in the middle of the text and encourage you to pause before routinely forging ahead. You have been presented with a lot of information to absorb and hopefully you have been given new ways to think about yourself and your relationship to food, your emotions, and your body. We are now ready to move from the realm of the physical and energetic body to explore your mind, or mental body. As you read on, I suggest that you consciously pace yourself so as not to become overwhelmed with the information and suggested tasks. This journey may start to feel like a laborious to-do list: revamping your diet, journaling your feelings, integrating exercise—and now meditation! It may be that you would like to take a break in even reading this book and instead backtrack and reinvest in some of the simple commitments suggested at the beginning of the book. I find that focusing on the level of the physical body can be very helpful when feeling overwhelmed because its concreteness grounds you in the real where you can take immediate action. When you are ready to move forward through the less tangible energies of emotion and into the realm of thought, pick up the book again. For it is here, in the fathomless realm of the mind, wherein lies your greatest human potential, as well as your most stunning fallibility.

Part Three

The Workings of Your Mind

Let's Dig In

We are now ready to enter the realm of your mind. Here we will explore yoga psychology with an intention to discern how this may help you further tap into the yoga of food using the power of your mind. I will continue introducing esoteric concepts and terms, but again I aim to keep them as simple as possible so that you can relate the ideas to your own experience. Chapter 5 explores the yogic understanding of the components of your psyche and the process of harnessing the power of your mind to further your well-being. Chapter 6 is about the Witnessing capacity of consciousness and explores your capacity to be objective about yourself—and how to use your objectivity to gain further insight into your patterns. We continue to stay grounded in the level of your personal self, though we are edging slowly toward embracing the larger spiritual awareness toward which yoga ultimately is oriented.

Chapter Five

Too Clever for Your Own Good (Manomaya Kosa)

When my interest in yoga was first developing, I staunchly resisted medi-tation. To be perfectly honest, although in theory I could understand its benefits, deep down I considered meditation an absurd waste of time. "Why would anyone in good conscience choose to sit and do nothing when there are so many productive things one could and should be doing?" So I would dutifully sit and breathe with others at yoga classes when so com-manded, secretly feeling extremely annoyed by the whole thing.

How did I, a determined non-meditator, transform into someone who is now peddling it as the next best thing to sliced, gluten-free bread? Let me reconstruct the path so you can understand how following the humble breadcrumbs of progressive change works. First, I began doing yoga. I felt a calling after my daughter was born. "I need to relax more," I said to my-self. So I took up yoga. It appeared to kill two birds with one stone—get a workout and chill out. Ironically, and this was not lost on me even at the time, I began practicing yoga in a very stressed out, obsessive way. I chose Bikram yoga, which is a series of static poses done in a very hot room. This style of yoga appealed to my obsessive nature due to its dependable structure and rigor. I was the one arriving almost late, at the front of the room, panting as I muscled into and fiercely held the various poses. I was also the one who more often than not skipped savasana, the final rest, at the end. So I took a step in the right direction ("I need to relax more. I'll try yoga.") and I brought my habitual patterns with me.

Let me pause here to discuss the role various teachers had in my development. The repetition of the reminders to breathe and to focus on the present, and the emphasis placed upon the importance of savasana in the integration of the yoga, were all extremely important to me, although at the time I apparently ignored most of this advice. I remember once when I was rather desperately holding dancer pose, which is quite challenging, gasping for breath but determined not to fall out, a male teacher gently advised that I try to breathe more slowly. "Look, buster, step away from the pose or you might get hurt!" I didn't actually say this and only part of me thought it. A deeper and wiser part of me registered his words. Another seed was cast.

The next step was deciding to do a yoga teacher training. I chose to do this mainly to develop my professional therapy practice—"Perhaps I'll teach my clients yoga rather than referring them to yoga," I thought to myself. The training gave me something much different than the professional development I was seeking. I met a wonderful group of people who exuded warmth, humor, and openness. I learned about yoga philosophy, the breath, and anatomy. Even more importantly, I felt supported by and included in a community. I was still staunchly opposed to meditation and felt safe enough to be honest about this. I remember toward the end of the training the leader saying gently to me, "I think you'll be surprised that you will be ready for meditation soon." She saw this potential in me before I did and made it a possibility on my horizon.

During the ten months of training, my physical energy was slowly declining, though I was not fully aware of it. My lack of awareness was mostly due to relating to my body primarily as a tool to obtain maximum pleasure and performance. Yes, I noticed that "it" (my body) was a little more tired and slow than before, but I was still able to get "it" to exercise regularly, so I wasn't overly concerned. About a month after the training ended, however, I became ill with a cold or some other seemingly benign virus. Little did I know that I had entered a ride that would take me on a frightening, at times apparently hopeless, journey into my body and eventually, my mind. The month of November, when I failed to recover, I chalked it up to being run-down. In December I felt a bit better, started my regular exercise routine, and fell back down into malaise. In January the same pattern continued. I went to my doctor, got some blood work and tested "normal." My throat felt inflamed and swollen. I was dizzy and tired. Toward afternoon, I would feel wretched. I went on, still expecting that I would get better. I would feel a little better for a few weeks, start exercising, and get clobbered. It was frightening and bewildering. In May, I decided to consult a naturopath. I went in terrified and defensive. My self-assessment had always been identified with being healthy, "healthier" than average. I had a lot of ego invested in this image and did not appreciate the fact that my precious identity was being challenged by none other than my very own body! Because of my defensiveness, it took several months to get any real traction in the recovery process, and real healing did not occur for quite a long time. The experience has given me a deep respect for the fragility and complexity of human health and its inextricable relationship to the mental and spiritual health. I came to discover that there was no one problem that needed to be "fixed." Healing has been ongoing and has involved several layers of letting go and opening up. The progress has been forward, but not linear. I realized about six months in, after suffering yet another setback, that I had to start addressing my mind. My entitlements and fears about health. My fixation on exercise and food. "Everything is mind," Baron Baptiste (the founder of a popular style of power yoga) croons in one of my regular yoga CDs. His statement had been echoing in my mind for a while. The seeds that had been planted by my yoga teacher training, by the umpteen yoga classes I had attended, by the Pema Chödrön CDs I had been steeped in, took root in the soil that had been upturned by my physical breakdown.

The point here is twofold. One, you must work with your mind if you expect to make sustained progress on the physical level. By exploring the patterns of your mind, you are given the data to understand how you create and perpetuate your own misery. In Iyengar's words, "We can go to a psychologist for advice, but in the end we are eternally obligated to fix our minds ourselves." You can't fix your mind if you are not familiar with its patterns and predilections. In order to develop this familiarity, you must quiet down enough to notice. The second point is that progress is not linear. Remember earlier when I discussed the common fantasy that you will go on a diet, take up yoga, go back to school, and wham, bam, you're new? Change does not work like that, at least not for most of us. No, instead we are like Hansel and Gretel, making our way along through a forest on the lookout for breadcrumbs leading us in the right direction. How do you know you are going in the right direction? That is a hard one to answer. But likely, as you go along, you will begin to contact more of your own intuitive wisdom about what is right for you. Also, you will reap results, subtle but real, in other areas of your life that will reinforce your commitment to meditation and better health. Each commitment builds upon itself and opens new doors and new possibilities. As you begin to feel what works for you and experience progress, you develop increasing trust in your intuition.

A Yogic Perspective on the Mind

Iyengar compares the mind to a lake. The surface ripples and waves are your everyday thoughts, often of a random or repetitive nature, "Oh, I've forgotten to buy the carrots." The author of *Light on Life* expounds on that thought, noting that your mind is very active, filled with useful and useless information alike. "…the point here is that a great many forces are constantly troubling the lake, muddying the waters, and agitating the surface." Traditionally in Classical Yoga, the body is addressed first in order to prepare for meditation. Balance in the body is not an endpoint—it is a prerequisite for being able to focus the mind. The real work of yoga, according to the Classical view, is to still the movement of the everyday mind. In Iyengar's words, "…a pure mind can reflect the beauty in the world around it, and when the mind is still, the beauty of the Self, or soul, is reflected in it." Now, this may sound like a rather highfalutin goal. "C'mon, sister," I hear you saying, "I just want to lose a few pounds." But really think about it. As long as you are wrapped up in your everyday mind, you are going to be bobbed around mercilessly by the whims of your appetite, your attractions, your aversions, and your fears (otherwise known as the kleshas). In essence, you must contact something larger inside yourself to sustain progress on the physical level.

According to yogic philosophy, there are four components of consciousness. The outermost layer is *manas*. This is the information processor, the tracker of the carrots, the chore list, the repository of jealousies, doubts, fears, and wishes. "What should I wear tonight?" "Boy, I've been looking fat lately." Manas is not bad: you need it to pay your taxes, get to work on time, and to remember the carrots. However, Iyengar cautions, "its nature is fickleness, unsteadiness, and inability to make productive choices," so it is not equipped to guide you in your life. *Chitta* is memory, will, and the decision-maker. *Buddhi* houses the part of you that learns to act on your own behalf and that has the capacity for insight and self-reflection. The "little voice" inside (intuition) that whispers what choice to make, usually when it's the harder choice, is buddhi. Iyengar makes a distinction between "cleverness," a quality of manas and "discrimination," a quality that belongs to buddhi. Cleverness often has to do with maximizing pleasure and avoiding pain, for example, finding a loophole in your taxes, while discrimination is making a choice in service of your personal growth. The deepest layer of consciousness is *ahamkara*, or the "I-maker," referring to the Egoic-self. Ahamkara masquerades as your true self, but this perception is misguided due to the ego's assumption that your individual self is separate and permanent. Aham-kara is preoccupied with attaining safety, pleasure, and permanence—futile preoccupations that fly in the face of the conditions of life on this planet, where uncertainty and change are the only constants. In Iyengar's words, "The Egoic self is an exhausting traveling companion, forever demanding that his caprices be pandered to, that his whims be obeyed (though he is never satisfied), and his fears be calmed (though they never can be)."

According to yogic philosophy, identifying too closely with Egoic-self/ ahamkara sets you up for suffering. As Iyengar described above, it is a futile quest to satisfy your ego-driven self. You may identify with the wisdom of his words if you stop to reflect on your own patterns and preoccupations. When you stop eating, do you seek to fill the space left by food with a new partner, a new dress, or a promotion? Remember how Sophie came to therapy because after reaching her weight-loss goal she no longer had that focus—and she started eating again? Notice your own restlessness, your fixations with what is wrong in your life, and your preoccupation with getting more of this (money, cake, love) and less of that (suffering, loneliness, insecurity). These incessant, circling preoccupations reveal the downfall of living a life driven by Egoic-self/ahamkara.

It is natural to confuse your true self with ahamkara. One might even argue that there is no such thing as a "true" self, so what are we even looking for? That issue goes far beyond the range of this discussion. What is perti-nent, and what I think most people can identify with, is the idea that we all share a small, Egoic-self that is concerned with short-term comforts and pleasures, and a larger, Wise-self that guides us toward more sustaining pur-suits. The crux of the matter is how closely identified you are with Egoic-self/ ahamkara and whether you have any contact with something larger and calmer in your mind. In my own daily life, my Egoic-self is concerned with what's for lunch, how many clients I have scheduled, and what so-and-so may think about me. My Wise-self is harder to define. I tune into this when

I am working meaningfully with a client, during meditation, and when I manage to contain myself and show restraint when faced with something inconvenient or offensive. This is just the beginning, of course. The idea is that by gradually devoting more and more time to pursuits that feed your Wise-self (buddhi), this capacity of your mind will grow. This deprives your Egoic-self (ahamkara) of sustenance, so that it gradually withers. This does not mean that you become ego-less, rather, your Egoic-self is no longer blindly leading the way and you are aware of how your tendencies toward selfishness or petty concerns interfere with your larger goals. The challenge is finding ways in our ego-driven society to feed your Wise-self and not get suckered into the pursuit of a new this or that to buy short-term "happiness." It is easier to do this once you start tasting the pleasures of living more in tune with Wise-self. The pleasure of insight, generosity, connection with another person, and doing the right thing, even when it is more difficult—like the enjoyment of a ripe peach, these deep pleasures are difficult to describe, though unmistakable when you experience them.

The following sections shall explore the manas, buddhi, and ahamkara in more depth to help you understand your mind in a different way, as well as help you understand how meditation may help you in your quest to become healthier. For ease of reading, from now on I shall refer to manas as "Clever-mind," buddhi as "Wise-self," and ahamkara as "Egoic-self." First we shall explore the "problems" associated with Clever-mind steering your boat. We discuss the short-lived nature of changes that are driven by your Egoic-self, specifically with regard to your weight-loss or health-enhancement efforts. Next, we'll explore how the delay between cause and effect presents a challenge when it comes to changing your health habits. Then we will be ready to move into the "solutions." First, we revisit the topics of impulse control and tapas/self-discipline (from chapter 4) with a focus on your mind's role in the development of these skills. Next, we explore the role of meditation in your growth process and go into some depth about how and, more importantly, why you should develop a meditation practice. Please hear this "should" in a kind, rather than controlling or moralistic tone. We will specifically address how meditation will help you understand, and eventually change, your relationship to food. The yoga of food involves making changes that are based on your greater well-being and not for the purposes of merely enhancing your image or creating a brand new, shiny "you" envisioned by your Egoic-self.

Reflections on the Workings of Your Mind

1. What is your reaction to the idea of working with your mind in order to address your issues with food and your body?

2. Can you relate the four components of consciousness to your experience of yourself? Can you differentiate between the chore-checking part of you (manas/Clever-mind); your memory, will, and decision-maker (chitta); the image you hold of yourself in your mind (ahamkara/Egoic-self); and the wiser part of your consciousness (buddhi/Wise-self)?

3. How much power does your Egoic-self have in your day-to-day life? What are the primary themes of your Egoic-self's concerns? Common examples are safety, status, or pleasure.

4. How often do you get in touch with your Wise-self? Your Wise-self has the capacity for compassion, generosity and understands how your own well-being is inextricably connected with others around you. What fosters your ability to contact this part of yourself? Examples are prayer, music, connection with others, art, and nature.

Who's in Charge?

When your Clever-mind (manas) is in the service of your Egoic-self (ahamkara), which is the common state of affairs, here is what happens. The cleverness of your everyday mind is used to accrue things that will hopefully solidify your Egoic-self's strength and stature. Feeling renewed after buying a new item is a good example of how your Egoic-self is buoyed up by material items. I remember a car salesman wooing me into a sale by telling me how professional and successful I would look in my new car. I am sorry to say that such crude tactics worked on me, but they did, and I bought a too-expensive car based on creating an image of myself as successful, rather than thinking about my actual needs. When you buy that new thing and see yourself as somehow different or enhanced by that thing, you are feeding your Egoic-self with fantasy wrought from the world of the material. The solid image you hold of yourself in your mind, and the common belief that a new this or that (car, house, relationship, body) will somehow make you "happy," is driven by fantasy that emanates from your Egoic-self. For me, identifying myself as "healthy" despite all the contrary evidence from my body is a good example of how the Egoic-self can fixate on solid beliefs that are not in sync with reality. Pushing myself to exercise when I didn't feel well shows the insanity of behavior motivated by the Egoic-self. In short, when your Egoic-self is in charge, you end up taking orders from a part of you that is misguided at best, and downright delusional at worst.

If you struggle with food or your body, you often experience a conflict between your wish to fit a particular image as "thin," "attractive," or "healthy" (images generated by your Egoic-self) and your reliance upon food to bind anxiety and soothe inner fragmentation. You can conceptualize this as a conflict between your Egoic-self ("I want to be thin," which is conceived as a solid, permanent state of being) and the straining of your Clever-mind for pleasure and avoidance of pain. If food is your primary soother, your Clever-mind is reflexively drawn to food. Your Egoic-self has little power to restrain the thrust of Clever-mind toward what it wants. Looking good for the wedding or fitting into a size 6 has no horsepower when facing the habitual groove of your Clever-mind, which over the years has reinforced your fixation on food for pleasure and relief from the toll of daily life. Due to the consequences of this habitual pattern, your Egoic-self resigns to labeling you as "fat," "lazy," or "a compulsive eater." When you do this, according to Iyengar, your Egoic-self has solidified you into a solid thing—"monolithic—like a great stone idol." This reduces your internal conflict and perpetuates the negative samskara/habitual pattern. After all, if you're "fat" or "lazy" (designations of your Egoic-self), then why bother? There can be an odd comfort in this resignation, even though it reinforces negative beliefs. Now you don't have to take the risk of making any uncomfortable changes. Your foreclosure, or collapse, dictates your future behavior, which is now just a repetition of the past. You justify your choices as inevitable due to genetics, secretly disdaining healthy eaters as "uptight." Or you may use the common "I just love to eat" statement to legitimize your foreclosure. Your Egoic-self has labeled you into a fixed thing ("fat") and then rationalizes your behavior based upon this label. The psychological term for this is cognitive dissonance—when your behavior is not consistent with your values ("I value health, but I am choosing to eat unhealthy food"), you manage this dissonance by rationalizing your inconsistent behavior, "Yes, I value health, but I just love to eat." For me, when I saw myself as "healthy" but felt terrible physically, I managed this cognitive dissonance by feeling like a victim and seeing myself as somehow inherently flawed or punished. At the time, I was unwilling to look at what habits might be reinforcing my ill health. When you are caught in the grips of such a refusal to get real with yourself, your Clever-mind will come up with a new diet or food plan that promises relief without requiring any substantive changes in your habits or priorities. In the case of fixation on weight loss, you fixate on a new diet (thought up by Clever-mind) to lose weight, while your Egoic-self perpetuates the belief that a new this or that—a body in this case—will create a new, acceptable self. This is a fantasy because "thin" or "fat" you will still be you and you will be sorely disappointed when you discover this to be the case. Your Egoic-self will shrug its shoulders and resign to shifting back to your old, ingrained identity as "fat" or "lazy." You feel relief along with disappointment because there is some odd comfort in knowing who you are, even if you don't like it very much. The Egoic-self enjoys certainty, even when the certainty is based on negative beliefs about yourself.

Wanda just had to lose weight for her daughter's wedding. (Remember Wanda, who eats compulsively in the evening?) Devastated by her divorce two years ago, she had cushioned herself from the serial blows of home foreclosure, transition to full-time work, and acceptance of her now ex-husband's chronic philandering with evening TV and sweet comfort foods. She had re-joined Weight Watchers to prepare for her daughter's wedding, where she anticipated having to endure her arrogant husband's smug ways and watch him flaunt his new relationship. She quickly lost twelve pounds. Then her night eating began to exert its sinister grip. "I wake up from my nap and just find myself in the kitchen." When she went to social gatherings, she described having to literally place herself away from the food tables or her arm, seemingly of its own volition, would automatically travel from food to mouth. As I previously mentioned, introducing some conflict into her experience by re-joining Weight Watchers was an important step for Wanda so that she was at least motivated to interrupt her pattern of mindless (buddhi-less) self-sabotage. However, doing it merely to look good at a wedding, to show her ex-husband that she was not "a loser," was inadequate fuel to motor a sustained shift in such ingrained, compulsive behavior. These motivation were generated from her Egoic-self's need to prove that she was "okay," or "not a loser," rather than emanating from something more stable and sustaining, like "I know that I am okay and I deserve to treat myself well." Motivation must come from your Wise-self, and a determination to act on your own behalf, in order to have any staying power.

One of the techniques Wanda began using to interrupt her evening eating was looking in the mirror and saying, "I can do this." This was effective for Wanda and signified a shift toward allying with something in herself that was deeper than the image in the mirror. For Wanda, affirming her competence, her ability to bear up to life and to her own impulses, was captured in this simple act of self-validation. We discussed other techniques, such as taking walks in the evening, journaling feelings, and painting to give her new ways of self-soothing. These techniques all give priority to the inside, which is invisible to others, rather than being motivated by the image seen by others, which is always in the service of enhancing the Egoic-self. Interestingly, when Wanda was able to withstand her compulsion to eat, she would feel a strong urge to call old boyfriends. Her Clever-mind, deprived of one satisfaction (food), strained for another thing to soothe and distract. Helping Wanda recognize this compulsive pattern of filling emptiness with "stuff" (in this case, old boyfriends are just fillers) was significant in her growth process.

As long as your Clever-mind is in service of your Egoic-self, you will get nowhere fast whether you are on a diet or not. When you are attempting to feel good merely to feel good, or to prove that you are good, your motivations will quickly wear thin. This is why you may have a string of "failed" diets in your past—they are all essentially the same! Iyengar suggests that "yoga points out how we generally react to the outside world by forming entrenched patterns of behavior that doom us to relive the same events endlessly, though in a superficial variety of forms and combinations." The Clever-mind keeps coming up with new strategies, but the issues remain the same. In order to break out of these samskaras/habitual patterns, you must harness of the power of your Wise-self. "The trick is to recognize which is which and then act on it. The paradox arises in that to train ourselves to achieve this, we have to start by doing a fair bit of what we don't want to do, and rather less of what we think we do," according to Iyengar. This may be translated as "No dessert unless you eat your vegetables." And the ongoing work is translating this punitive tone into a voice of nurturance and self-care. The yoga of food is about making food choices with a tone of nurturance. This does not mean being "perfect" or impeccable with regard to your food choices. It does mean being mindful and nurturing and allowing the answer to the gentle question "Is this good for me?" to guide your choices.

Reflections on Your Dominant Mind

1. Are your wishes to lose weight and be healthier in the service of your Egoic-self or your Wise-self? How can you tell? If you

are losing weight for an event in order to impress others, this is a sure sign that your Egoic-self is calling the shots. If you are changing your eating habits because you are tired of the pain poor food choices have created in your life and your body, then you are acting more in the service of your Wise-self.

2. How do you feel about the idea of training yourself to do more of what you don't want to do and less of what you do want to do? Do you believe that practicing new, sometimes difficult behaviors consistently over time will result in you actually wanting more of what is good for you?

The Delay Between Action and Consequence

Iyengar points out that due to evolution, the delay between action and consequence has been considerably extended compared to days past. In the old days, Clever-mind, which functions in a binary way (repeat pleasure/avoid pain), was well suited to deal with threats such as typhoid or cholera. "Drink contaminated water on Monday, sick on Tuesday, dead on Wednesday." Since the calculus of Clever-mind is exceedingly simple ("pleasure good/ pain bad"), it is equipped to successfully cause you to avoid the contaminated water. By contrast, "We nearly all recognize that there is some connection between the way we live and such illnesses as cancer, heart disease, and arthritis, yet since the process of decline is so gradual and the deadly payoff so long deferred, we find it terribly difficult to make the necessary reforms in our habits of life, even if, at one level, we are actually longing for them." Iyengar goes on to say, "The longer the delay between the primary action/ inaction and its secondary effect, the more tempted we are to prevaricate, lie to ourselves, refuse to jump our fences, and take the downhill path." So now you are dealing with eat cheeseburgers regularly and get heart disease in twenty years. Or eat junk food today and feel uncomfortable at the wedding next month. Clever-mind is not designed to process this kind of information usefully, particularly when your energy and emotions are focused on getting you through the day. This chasm between cause and effect is where we so often lose our bearings and go astray.

The fact that this pattern is so deeply human, so stunningly predictable, can give you heart along the path. It's not just you. It's not just me. "Hence, we must train ourselves to do actions now that we would rather not do in order to reap consequences that we desire at some later point in the future. Do something now that would be easier not to do (math homework instead of TV or get up an hour earlier for some yogasana practice) and reap the benefit a bit later. Repeat it often enough and harvest the compound interest as the future unrolls." Do you notice how Iyengar's advice is somewhat repetitious? Do something now that is hard and get the benefit later. Isn't that the advice your mother gave you? Or should have given you. Rebelling against this rule of reality does you no good.

Cindy recently had a hysterectomy. She made the decision due to having been quite compromised by pelvic discomfort for several years. After the surgery, she was beside herself with fear regarding her healing process and the possibility of a negative outcome. Her biggest fear was prolapse of her bladder, and she knew that carrying some extra weight in her abdomen made this outcome more probable. We addressed her fears in a session not long after the surgery. Addressing her feelings without dramatization, which would add to the klesha/obstacle of fear in a way that she would find overwhelming, was important. Yet it was also important to not minimize, or dilute, her grasp on the very real potential consequences to her current health choices. During the session, I reminded Cindy that she has the power of choice in her life and that she did not need to be a victim of her fear and the eventual physical manifestation of this. Cindy wept during the session as she confronted her fears about living life without the ready comfort of food. "I just want to eat and die young," she sobbed at one point. Interestingly, the next week she walked in looking much brighter and lighter, having just made some changes in her eating habits.

Go figure. Despair and determination are more closely juxtaposed than you might think. There is something invigorating about facing life on life's terms, coming to terms with despair, and making the decision to not succumb to its downward pull. Cindy's case illustrates this key fact—that swinging between the extremes of motivation and collapse is not unusual. Growth occurs when the polarities become less extreme and the delay between progression and regression diminishes, as I will discuss later on.

Another less dramatic, but still quite relevant illustration of the empowerment wrought from facing the consequences of health choices is illustrated by Mandy. Mandy is a former homecoming queen. Her hundred-pound-plus weight gain was the slow creep that occurs for those who just "love" food and no longer participate in team sports of their youth. Now in her late thirties and highly uncomfortable due to extra weight, she made a decision to reform. About two months in to her new commitment to health, she was having a moment of temptation and confided to a coworker her strong desire for a cheeseburger. Expecting commiseration and collusion, she was shocked when her coworker replied, "Okay then, go get a cheeseburger, go home, and take your clothes off and eat it in front of the mirror." Wow! This shot of reality was significant enough for Mandy to go on to lose eighty pounds. She came to see me when she was floundering in her weight-loss efforts long after this comment from her coworker. Though the comment still rang in her mind, it had lost its power to motivate her. This illustrates how easy it is to lose sight of the consequences of our daily behavior, the inevitable problem with the delay between cause and effect that Iyengar describes. Another problem with her coworker's motivational tip was that it focused too much on the outside (the image in the mirror, or her Egoic-self) and not enough on the inside, and the regretful feelings Mandy had about not taking good care of her body.

It is through discrimination, which is guided by your Wise-self/buddhi, that you begin to make choices that are truly in your best interest and aligned with the reality of life in a body. The power of discrimination must be based on love for yourself, which is generated by your Wise-self. When you struggle with your weight, using discrimination has to do with entering the inner domain of your body and making choices based on your health, the actual reality of your body/annamaya kosa, rather than image that is perpetuated by your Egoic-self, or the momentary whims of your Clever-mind. When you make this step, you harness the cleverness of your Clever-mind to create future health and well-being. Clever-mind is now in the service of Wise-self. This shift requires you to bring some discipline (tapas!) to the perpetual straining of Clever-mind for pleasure. And this brings us back to the topic of impulse control.

Reflections on Action and Consequence in Relations to Your Health

1. Reflect on what your health will be like in ten, twenty, or thirty years if you continue your current patterns. Do you tend to avoid these considerations? Is this too much reality?

2. Again, reflect on your relationship to the idea of "discipline." Does the word evoke harshness or kindness?

Learning to Act on Your Own Behalf— A Buddhist Perspective on Impulse Control

Your daily thoughts are full of "shoulds" and judgments. These can be quite toxic and not at all helpful in the change process. In fact, "shoulds" and judgments can feel like hammers that you use against yourself in a way that breaks down your self-esteem and diminishes your motivation. But sometimes these seemingly toxic thoughts contain important information. Perhaps you could benefit from more exercise or a change in your diet. Perhaps your current habits in these areas are causing you pain. The challenge is to act on this knowledge from a place of self-affirmation without the toxic effects of judgment. The key to doing this is determined by whether the "shoulds" are emanating from Wise-self or Egoic-self. As discussed above, if the "shoulds" are in the service of creating a nicer, shinier, more acceptable you (your Egoic-self), they will be no match for the habitual, pleasure driven

Clever-mind (remember, Clever-mind is designed to maximize pleasure and has little grasp of long-term consequences). However, if the "shoulds" are in the service of Wise-self, if you really are aware of how your health habits are causing you suffering, then you are aligned with your own best interest and impulse control feels somehow "right," rather than depriving.

After her daughter's wedding, Wanda's efforts toward reforming her health habits began to falter again. "What's it going to take for me to get this?" This was a question she often repeated in our sessions when she was lamenting her eating habits. "I ate again last night," she informed me one day. "After dinner I ate twenty of those mini peanut-butter cups, a granola bar, and a bowl of cereal." She shook her head in disgust, yet somehow seemed distanced from her regret. A few weeks later, Wanda informed me that she had been diagnosed with type 2 diabetes. She had been aware of this consequence for a while, having been "pre-diabetic" for a few years. But a quiet transformation took place. She stopped eating sugar. She stopped talking about sugar. I asked her how she was doing with her eating habits in a session about a month after her diagnosis. "It's just not an option," she stated matter-of-factly. She is not happy about this and admits that it's "hard," but she has accepted it. Her Wise-self is calling the shots now, and Clever-mind has quit complaining and bargaining.

Pema Chödrön, a Tibetan Buddhist nun who writes and lectures on the power and process of meditation, provides a helpful framework for developing impulse control in her lecture series, "Getting Unstuck." Her formula goes like this: *"Recognize. Relax. Refrain. Resolve."* Let's break it down and see how a Buddhist perspective can enhance your understanding of how working with the mind can facilitate positive changes in your body.

"Recognize": This is where the process of establishing more intimacy with your patterns comes in. You say to yourself, "Aha! here I am again craving a quick fix of carbohydrates when I am feeling depleted in the face of afternoon demands." It is important to note here that this requires a mild dissociation from your experience—you are not just craving chips, you are noticing yourself craving chips. The other important point is that this recognition is not

used as a hammer to beat yourself with: "Dammit, I just had lunch. Why the hell am I wanting to eat again?" The concept of mitri, unconditional friendliness toward the self, is vital here. Mitri neutralizes the judgment that so often accompanies self-recognition.

"Relax": This is way to bring mitri/self-love into your direct experience. We habitually tighten up when confronted with conflict, be it from the outside or on the inside. Inner conflict, although unseen by others, is still very real. Your stomach clenches, your jaw tightens, and your shoulders hunch. You will not give in. This restraint can only last so long because it's exhausting. When a client informs me that they are "white-knuckling it," I always worry. In contrast, when you are cultivating intimacy with your patterns, and more acceptance of your cravings and impulses, you gradually develop ease with the rise and fall of your habitual cravings. Instead of fighting your hungers, you breathe into them, name them, and allow them without necessarily acting on them. They no longer have power over you because you are in a relationship of non-resistance with them.

"Refrain": This word brings a subtle difference than the word "resist," which connotes strong-arming yourself into good behavior. Refrain means setting a mindful boundary that is in your own best interest and respecting this boundary even if you don't necessarily like it—just like Wanda demonstrated above, firmness without harshness. Refrain also has a double meaning, a repeating measure in a piece of music. Think of refraining as a repeating measure of restraint that you bring to your daily life.

"Resolve": You may not find this one to be particularly inspiring. It is tied to the fact that when you are working with deep habitual patterns/samskaras, you do not refrain once, twice, or even one hundred times. Rather, you resolve to repeat this process of self-recognition, relaxation, and refraining over and over and over again. The good news is, as with practicing a piece of music, this process will become easier and easier over time until it becomes a graceful, seemingly effortless flow in your daily life.

This formula is more conceptual than practical. Meaning, if you are poised before the cupboard, hand reaching for the Oreo cookies, it is unlikely that you will say to yourself, "Now what was that again, am I supposed to refrain, or was that relax? What the heck...?" Rather, this formula is meant to illustrate a basic attitude that you begin cultivating toward your less laudatory impulses. The basic attitude is one of acceptance and mindfulness. You are committing to acting on your own behalf and willing to evaluate your behaviors based upon this basic tenet. "Is this good for me?" is your new refrain.

———————

Janice had joined a medically supervised weight-loss program and was fifty pounds into a journey she deemed to be two hundred pounds total. Egoic-self likes solid numbers, and though there is nothing "wrong" with this, it does not have a lot of staying power when thrust up against the power of Clever-mind's attraction to comfort. A few months into the program, Janice found herself triggered by the group leader. Janice is the meticulous employee with the messy home and a body that she once described to me as "a garbage disposal." As a child, she was the apple of her father's eye. Her father was a cruel, primitive man who alternatively comforted and punished her with food. He would bring her Happy Meals to help her through the school day, imprinting her with a deep sense of security tied to fast food. At another time, as you may recall, he forced her to eat a whole can of chocolate syrup when she accidentally put too much on her ice cream. These mixed messages about food and love were deeply confusing to Janice, who now used food to both comfort and punish herself as an adult. We learn to treat ourselves as we were treated. When Janice was in junior high, her father decided she needed to exercise. He would sit in his armchair and force her through a series of calisthenics on a daily basis as he sat comfortably and imperiously observing her. Janice found the experience humiliating and enraging. Afterward, she would go to her bedroom and stuff herself with her stash of junk food. She'd show him! She exerted the only power she had at the time. This story illustrates how in our own psyches the deep traumas continue to repeat and shape our experience until we are able to fully process them.

Janice had to miss a few meetings at the weight-loss program due to a preplanned vacation followed by an unexpected work meeting. Participation required weekly weigh-ins and group attendance. Members were allowed to miss one session but would be dismissed from the program if they missed more than that. Janice was diligently working the program and expected the leader to recognize her dedication and not hold her to the letter of the law (or program rules). The leader granted the additional absence, but only on the condition that Janice come in twice that week to make up for her second missed session. Janice was furious. She complied with the seemingly arbitrary rule and sat through the required meeting with unconcealed anger toward the leader. Janice was terrified of her own anger and was usually an assiduously congenial and accommodating person. And here she was, openly defiant and outraged in a public arena! Following this incident, Janice ate like a demon had been unleashed inside her. She ate a whole gallon of Cold Stone Creamery ice cream in a day, "And I don't even like ice cream!" she later recounted.

Janice found this experience deeply instructive about the magnitude of rage she feels for arbitrary authority and her use of food to rebel. She "recognized" herself at a deep level. She was able to "relax" into this self-recognition and get back on track with the program and the group leader. Relaxation is signified by her not beating herself up for her lapse, but rather being interested in what it had to teach her. She "refrained" from the compulsion to continue her self-destructive behavior. Her "resolve" to stay with the process was strengthened by this ordeal and the insight she had wrought from it. In this scenario, Janice was initially at the mercy of her Clever-mind, which strained for relief from painful feelings of shame and anger by the use of an ingrained, dysfunctional behavior. Her Egoic-self was tied to this behavior as a way to assert her autonomy, even if it was at her own peril. "I'll show her," her Egoic-self chimed in, egging on her self-destructive behavior. Eventually, she was able to harness the power of her Wise-self and use this experience to deepen her commitment to her growth process. Her Egoic-self's fixation on the number (200 pounds!) was no longer the most prominent motivator. Numbers lose their power as we engage more fully with the energy of growth.

Reflections on Impulse Control

1. Do you habitually try to "control" yourself when you are on a diet? How can you relax when you feel tempted to sabotage your well-being?

2. Can you relate to Janice's self-sabotage? Can you see the importance of allying with yourself even after "bad" behavior?

3. Can you imagine recognizing your impulses to eat, get angry, or act out in a self-defeating way, without acting on the impulse?

4. Further consider your relationship to self-discipline/tapas. Does the word "refrain" resonate with you as a gentler way to conceptualize limits?

How Meditation Can Help

Your Clever-mind/manas is not bad. Remember, your Clever-mind is the part of you that takes care of life's little details to help you solve everyday problems. In fact, it can be of great help to you as you commit to taking better care of yourself. Clever-mind will help you with your food choices and will help you find time to fit meditation into your busy schedule. In order to harness the "cleverness" of your mind, however, you must strengthen contact with your Wise-self/buddhi. Buddhi is the part of you that helps make decisions based upon your long-term needs. Hence, when you refrain from the gustatory temptations that are part of our everyday life here in the West, you will not be storing up feelings of deprivation and martyrdom because your restraint is emanating from your conviction that this is truly in your best interest. You begin to realize that when you set boundaries and make wise choices (exercise impulse control), you just plain feel better. You realize that what may feel good going down in the moment has effects you will have to live with for many hours, and if you do it over and over, it will have effects you will need to deal with in many years. So when Clever-mind says, "You should (or shouldn't) eat this," or "You should exercise," these directives are not heard as commands to make you into a better object or product (in the service of your Egoic-self). Neither are you as vulnerable to Clever-mind's intention to make you as comfortable as possible in the short term, regardless of the long-term consequences. Instead, Clever-mind is now increasingly allied with your Wise-self and its directives are aimed to help you stay on a path that is more aligned with reality and your own well-being. So when your Clever-mind says, "You shouldn't have eaten that," you do not use this as a stick to beat yourself with, but rather as information to help you make better choices tomorrow. In this case, your Clever-mind is in dialogue with your Wise-self, as you realize that the choice you made did not necessarily serve your greater aspirations for health and enhanced well-being.

By training your mind, you can learn how to differentiate the thoughts that serve your Egoic-self from the thoughts that serve your Wise-self. By focusing your attention, you strengthen the attentional wiring of your brain. You also become more familiar with the trains of thought populating your inner world. Daniel Siegel, a psychiatrist who advocates meditation as an adjunct to therapy, uses the metaphor of lifting a weight when he describes learning meditation. He uses this metaphor to explain how the very act of bringing your attention back to your breath when it wanders is the lifting of the weight. Analogous to actual weight lifting, you don't curse at yourself and accuse yourself of being irredeemable when you bring the weight down during a set. No, you understand that putting the weight down is integral to the process of building muscle and you lift the weight back up. So it is with meditation. Your mind wanders (puts down the weight of focused attention) and you bring it back to your breath (you lift the weight). The very act of noticing that your attention has wandered and subsequently bringing it back to your breath is what constitutes the practice. And it's okay if your attentional muscles are very flabby at first. How could they not be? This is the very reason why you are practicing! Through consistent practice, you learn to differentiate between Clever-mind in the service of function, "I need to buy carrots" or in the service of Egoic-self, "I need to lose weight before I can take up yoga," and Clever-mind in the service of Wise-self, "I will feel better if I order the salad," or "I should meditate today so that I stay consistent with my goal to follow through on commitments." Over time, strengthening your attention builds enormous internal power because it allows you to more consciously choose where you want your attention to go, which of your thoughts you want to feed and which you don't. Do you want to be incessantly preoccupied with a biological need of your body? Or with changing the shape and size of your body? Having these thoughts is both your choice and not your choice. It is not your choice in the sense that you cannot control your thoughts—they run of their own accord. However, you can begin to control the volume button on your thoughts and grow in your capacity to disregard thoughts that are not useful and even defy thoughts when they are destructive. Meditation will help you learn to use the controls in your mind with more acuity and discrimination.

How to Meditate

Describing how to meditate is a bit like describing how to watch paint dry. Sit down, choose an object to focus on, breathe. It is apparently such a simple thing to do. There are no fancy bells or whistles, no colorful control panel to master. It is a practice of subtlety. Because the practice is so subtle, because you will not lose weight or burn calories, earn money, or have anything tangible to show for your efforts, motivating yourself to practice it will likely be difficult at first. But, really, this is the essence of why the practice is so good for you. It is a deep affirmation of Self. It is an affirmation of your right to "Be," regardless of your output or mastery. It is also an affirmation of the importance of your interior world, as opposed to what you look like and what you have to show for yourself. The interior world is a mysterious landscape, full of incongruity, drama, and tedium. It takes time to familiarize yourself with this terrain because it is so different from the terrain of daily life, which is often populated by loud noises, bright lights, and "reality" shows. Karen Horney, a well-known psychoanalyst from days past (way before insurance companies), stated that the first goal of psychotherapy was to get the patient to become interested in him or herself. This idea of getting interested in yourself, as opposed to "fixing" yourself, nicely frames an initial goal of meditation.

I will describe some of the basic practicalities and technicalities of starting a meditation practice. First, choose the place where you will practice. This is important, but not to the point that you should let it stand in the way of getting started. I have had clients wait to start a practice because they want to create a peaceful room in their home, but first they have to clean the room out, decorate it, and buy a fountain to create ambiance. This is a delay tactic! There is nothing wrong with creating a nice place in your home, but your practice is going to be about sitting with the messiness of your thoughts, and if you are fantasizing that a nice room with a fountain will make this any easier, then you are fantasizing. So just find a quiet place in your home. I suggest not using your bed for the simple reason that your bed is associated with sleep, and meditation is not something you want to associate with unconsciousness. Also, it is better to have a firm place to sit. If you have back trouble or some other physical problem, sit with your spine straight in chair. You may choose to sit on a cushion on the floor if you can do this comfortably. Sitting against a wall or a piece of furniture can help with your posture if you choose to sit on the floor.

In this form of meditation, you use your breath as the focus for your attention. Breathe through your nose, counting lightly on the exhale. You may keep your eyes slightly open or close them if you prefer. I suggest that you experiment with different techniques to focus on your breath and see what feels right. You may count your breaths, starting at 1 and counting to 10 or 20 before returning to 1. When you forget where you are, and you will (the first lesson of meditation is that your mind will wander), you start over at 1. Alternatively, you may focus on the sensation of air entering your nostrils or on the movement of your chest or abdomen. You can set a timer or use a clock and set a reasonable goal, such as 5 minutes if you are totally new to meditation. I suggest doing your practice twice a day at the beginning in order to acclimate yourself to the technique and the very idea of sitting quietly doing "nothing." After about a week or two of sitting for 5 minutes twice a day, you may double the time to 10 minutes twice a day. In another week, you are ready for 15 minutes. You may stay at 15 minutes for a while, several weeks if you wish. You may choose to shorten your meditation if you find yourself dreading, avoiding, or resenting the practice. The trick here is calibrating your practice so that you are not sabotaging yourself by making it too overwhelming, which increases the odds that you will quit. The eventual goal that I suggest you work toward is 20 minutes to 30 minutes a day. Longtime meditators have told me that 30 minutes is a good baseline because it takes at least 10 minutes to quiet your mind and get to a deeper level of awareness. But the biggest thing is to do what you can and respect your own schedule and needs. You don't need to take a big portion (30 minutes) just because someone else has that much. Experiment to see what feels right for you and stick with that. The yoga of food helps you begin to assess your needs and meet them respectfully in all areas of your life.

Steps for Developing Your Meditation Practice

1. Find a place to meditate in your home. Make sure that you are comfortable in the place you have chosen. Use a chair that will assist you in sitting up straight if you have back problems or use a cushion on the floor if you can keep your spine straight. Have a clock that you can see or use a timer to keep track of your minutes.

2. Decide when you will practice and for how long. I suggest starting with 5 minutes twice a day and building from there.

After a week, try doubling to 10 minutes twice a day. After another week, go for 15 minutes. You will be surprised that this amount becomes doable, perhaps even something that you look forward to.

3. Keep a journal logging your practice. It is helpful to note your reactions, especially any benefit you notice from the practice. Reflect on why you are meditating and what your goals for practicing are. I suggest keeping your goals very limited and focused on showing up, not on achieving some miraculous state of mind. Showing up on your cushion and learning to sit with whatever state you are in is the first goal of meditation.

4. Notice how much you think about food when you meditate. Notice your response to noticing how much you think about food. Relax your judgment and practice just noticing.

Beneath Your Chattering Mind

You must enter this new endeavor with a commitment to develop patience with yourself. Your mind will wander. A lot. This is not due to a character defect. Rather, it is the nature of your Clever-mind to chatter. You can consider it like a CB radio, broadcasting over the airwaves particular stations that you are tuned into. Underlying your particular choice of broadcasting is your Egoic-self and at times your Wise-self. As you gain more facility with the practice, you will have more discrimination regarding the airwaves you wish to broadcast.

At the beginning, meditation is a process of learning to not identify so much with your thoughts and to instead watch your thoughts. Through observing your thoughts, you get to know yourself better. You begin to understand your Egoic-self's preoccupations better. What beliefs about yourself are you attached to? Are you often rehashing interchanges with other people? Are you thinking about your children? Your dog? What you will wear that day? What you will eat that day? All of the above? You will begin to notice themes to the thoughts that come up most frequently. Certain thoughts are more repetitive and captivating than others. It may seem like an odd concept, but you are actually using meditation to get to know yourself better. Many of us think that we know ourselves quite well, after all, we are "ourselves," right? But actually, we are often quite blind to our most prominent issues. You may have a vague idea that you have "control" issues, but you need some distance from being caught up in your thoughts so that you can see yourself more clearly without all the noise. You may discover that your "control" issues are masking a great deal of fear or shame. You learn this about yourself as you "watch" your thoughts, which incessantly hover around social interactions and whether or not you said the right thing, or what so-and-so may think about you. As you "see" this recurrent theme, you begin to recognize the limitations of this preoccupation and you have more distance from this concern in your daily life.

Meditation cultivates distance from the immediacy of your thoughts, you see yourself thinking rather than being captivated by the drama of your thoughts and then mindlessly acting them out. For example, with regard to food, in your daily life you may find yourself "starving" in the middle of a big project at work. Intent on finishing the project, you go to the candy machine and quickly scarf something down to get you through the project. During meditation, you may notice your thoughts repetitively going to food after considering all the things you have to do that day. "Hmmm ... ," you may say to yourself after some time on the cushion, "I seem to use food to deal with pressure." Or "I tend to eat when I really need to rest." Knowing this about yourself on a more conscious level enhances your ability to choose how you will respond to these ingrained patterns. You may choose to eat well at lunch knowing that you are under a lot of pressure in the afternoon, and you don't forget to pack a protein-rich snack to see you through the rough spots. Or you choose to take a break and lie down on floor for fifteen minutes in the afternoon. When you notice your mind going to food, you say, "Oh, there you go again," with a gentle smile.

One of the biggest misconceptions about meditation is that you are doing it to relax. If you are under this impression, I give you about a week before you cast the whole endeavor aside and declare yourself a lost cause. Meditation will not relax you, at least not at the beginning. In fact, it can be quite the opposite because you come face to face with your internal turmoil without traffic, screaming kids, or unreasonable spouses to blame it on. No, it's just you and your thoughts, up close and personal. In your daily life, you may swim in negative thoughts without even being aware of the milieu. Like a fish swimming in murky water, you don't even know it's murky until you emerge for a moment and look in your fishbowl from the top—"Aha," you may say, "what a cesspool!" Because you are not so identified with the "rightness" of your thoughts, you are able to look at them with more discernment and objectivity. You notice that you tend to be very negative without judging yourself, but instead with an eye toward understanding your conditioning more fully.

Currently there is a movement toward "positive thinking." People are diligently making gratitude lists and wrenching their miserable minds into a state of thankfulness. This movement was epitomized by the movie *The Secret*, which promulgated the law of attraction—think it, and it shall be so. Obsessed with negativity? Then you are creating your own bad luck. In my opinion, this line of reasoning can be somewhat dangerous. I have nothing against gratitude, mind you. However, suppressing your negativity and labeling it "bad" is no shortcut to gratitude. Rather, unconditional positive regard for yourself, including your negativity, is important to cultivate. The intent is counterintuitive, especially in our problem-solving culture. The intention that I am describing is not to change or fix the "problem" of your negativity, but rather to grow more familiar with its edges. For me, this means getting curious about my fears and doubts. "What is this worry? Where is the tightness? What is the fear?" By letting go of your agenda to "fix" yourself, you create an atmosphere of acceptance for yourself that goes a long way toward diluting your negativity.

Reflections on Your Chattering Mind

1. Do you notice prominent themes in the thoughts that your mind replays during your meditation practice?

2. What information does this give you about yourself? How might this be useful for you in your growth process?

3. How much negativity do you notice in your primary thought patterns? Are there prominent themes to your worries? Examples of common themes are money, health concerns, or social status.

Food for Thought

Meditation strengthens your ability to be in the present moment, in the reality of your present, breathing body. Focusing your mind on your breath is both a literal coming back to your body as well as grounding yourself in the here and now. Most people have a very hard time being in the present—Clever-mind is dutifully checking off the chore list, planning dinner, or rehashing something from yesterday or ten years ago. When I meditate now, I often experience moments when my thoughts are less persistent, and I feel as though my consciousness drops in to my body. I am aware of a warm buzz of internal energy, my breath feels fuller, and I experience my whole body for a few moments. This is more than a "feel good" moment. Rather, it is an integrative moment—integrating my body into my awareness so that I am in the present and in my body rather than caught up in the chatter of my Clever-mind. This is powerful because when you experience this level of integration during meditation, you will be more aware of the disconnect when you are hijacked by your thoughts in your day-to-day life. When you are far from home, you forget what home was like. Meditating reintroduces you to being at home in your body, as opposed to panting and obsessing, or robotically maneuvering your way through life. Experiencing this feeling for 30 seconds, 2 minutes, 10 minutes, and eventually 30 minutes when you are meditating makes it more likely you will recognize when you are not present in your body during your daily life. When you can recognize this, then you can relax and recalibrate—that is, you can self-regulate. This greatly mitigates the power that reflexive patterns have over your behavior.

Let's look at this in relation to overeating. The reflexive need to binge, or self-soothe with food, arises from a place of stress and disintegration. You are not grounded in your body or in the present moment. Current brain science allows us to visualize what this state might look like on an MRI. Likely, your brain stem and limbic system (specifically the amygdala, which regulates fear) are lit up and your prefrontal cortex (which regulates higher level awareness) looks rather gray (no blood flow). Due to your habitual pattern/samskara of regulating stress with food, your primitive brain says, "Me must eat!" Out the window go your aspirations for better health and well-being, ideals housed in your prefrontal cortex. These ideals just plain don't exist for you at the moment because your prefrontal cortex is offline. Well, if you need more convincing regarding the benefits of meditation, here it is! Meditation actually strengthens your prefrontal cortex. Yes, quite literally, MRIs prove that people who meditate have a thicker prefrontal cortex, which indicates more neurons and more myelination, according to Daniel Seigel and Jack Kornfield, creators of *The Mindful Brain*. Consider meditation a workout for your brain. As you "work out" your prefrontal cortex during meditation, you strengthen its wiring, making it more likely that you will eventually be able to shift from a place of primitive self-soothing to a higher level of awareness. This means your prefrontal cortex is able to pipe in, "I am feeling really raw right now. How can I take care of myself in a way that is not self-destructive?" You are able to integrate your higher aspirations for good health and well-being even when you are at your wits end. Wise-self/buddhi is online!

Reflections on Food for Thought

1. Do you have a hard time being in the present moment? How might this be related to your food issues? Notice how "present" you are when you are eating. Are you tasting your food? Taking time to swallow? Try putting your fork down between bites.

2. When you meditate do you become more aware of your body? What do you notice?

3. Can you relate to the idea of being hijacked by your primitive brain when you overeat? Does conceptualizing it this way help with your shame about overeating?

The yoga of food has to do with relating to food with more conscious, loving intention. We started this journey by helping you to appreciate the materiality and physicality of your body with heightened awareness. This is the realm of the annamaya kosa. Our work in this area involved helping you harness the power of cause and effect by helping you to choose higher quality food with which to nourish your body. We then moved on to explore the role of emotions and energy in your food choices and explored how the physical practice of yoga could be of service in finding alternative, health-enhancing ways to calm jangled energy patterns. This is the realm of the pranamaya kosa. Next we stepped into the realm of your mind and addressed the role your thoughts have in your creation of self. This is the manomaya kosa. Through-out this journey, we have stayed in the realm of your personal self. The phi-losophy of yoga guides you toward grasping your interconnection with oth-ers, and ultimately with the universe, and hence brings you toward spiritual development. This book is not meant to take you toward this level of yoga. However, we are now approaching a greater awareness that reaches beyond mere self-awareness. We are set to explore your capacity to have insight, or what is also referred to as your Witnessing consciousness. The next chapter explores the process of developing your capacity for a more objective level of self-awareness, called Witnessing. We are still at the level of your personal self, but moving incrementally toward a higher level of consciousness, which, don't forget, is the larger purpose of yoga.

Chapter Six

Getting Closer to Your Wisdom Body (Vijnanamaya Kosa)

Remember the story I told you earlier about my issues with being late? What allowed me to tell that story? Well, it is my ability to stand to the side and watch myself as if I am an observer. When I do this, there is no judgment. Instead, I am relating the facts, and if I wished, I could get more into it, analyzing the reasons for this persistent behavior, what I may get out of it, why I might have developed this in the first place... At some point, this analysis becomes irrelevant and it's time to make a change. However, we cannot underestimate the importance of this ability to look at ourselves objectively. It is what makes us human and what makes us capable of change. When was the last time your dog mentioned to you that he really needs to stop wolfing his food down or that he realizes that his habit at staring at you when you are eating is extremely intrusive and annoying? Exactly. And that's why Fido is likely not going to change his habits any time soon.

The Witness (which is known as the "observing ego" in Western psychological terminology) is the part of you that sees yourself from a more objective view. It emanates from buddhi and fuels your capacity to act on your own behalf. The Witnessing capacity of your consciousness is extraordinarily important in the process of change because it allows you to see your patterns and their consequences. I will capitalize the Witness to indicate its stature in your consciousness and also to convey the idea that there is an "otherness" to it. By otherness, I mean that the Witness is the interface between you and universal intelligence. As Iyengar reminds us, "…we must begin to understand that our individual intelligence, though an essential rudder to guide us, is merely a puny offshoot of cosmic intelligence (mahat), which is the organizing system of the universe." The Witness as I am using the term is firmly embedded within the personal self and so does not rise to the spiritual level of the anadamaya kosa/bliss body. It is edging in on the vijnanamaya kosa/wisdom body, which links you to universal intelligence and therefore gives this capacity in your consciousness so much horsepower.

The following sections will describe ways to enhance your access to this extraordinary aspect of your Being. We remain anchored in the personal self, and therefore are not fully entering the realm of the vijnanamaya kosa. That remains for you to access more deeply as you remain on the path of yoga.

Let us start our exploration by utilizing Iyengar's understanding of this higher capacity of our mind. "Intelligence has two overriding characteristics. First, it is reflexive; it can stand outside the self and perceive objectively, not just subjectively. When I am being subjective, I say I hate my job. When I am being objective, I say I have the skills to get a better job."

In this quote, Iyengar points out the difference between the sentiments, "I hate my job," and "I have the skills to get a better job." When you are in a purely subjective mode, you are caught up in your "story," captive of the predetermined plot line, which pulls you inexorably into its particular logic.

You hate your job, you are trapped, doomed to be a failure … The plot takes on more momentum as it unfolds, pulling you along in its tide. This is likely how you live out your relationship with food. You hate your body, have no willpower, and are consequently helpless and incapable of change.

In contrast, a more objective view steps outside of the predetermined plot and risks changing the story line. You must have the ability to see beyond the concrete "realities" of the present, of your particular job (or body) in order to become more objective. It is as if you step away from the sweep of your emotions and habitual reactions to a situation and Witness yourself through a wider lens. You are both you and not you—you are watching yourself with some interest and objectivity. Your perspective shifts from a tight, constricted lens to a slight distance, where you can take stock of the details with a more dispassionate vision. This allows you to make a decision regarding how you can best cope with the situation. In relation to food, the light bulb goes on and you see clearly that you have choices in the matter.

Let me illustrate this shift in perspective with an example from my fledgling meditation practice. Recently, I was struggling with a situation regarding parenting my daughter that gives me a great deal of pain. It was a Sunday and I was doing my best to bear up, however, my mind kept mulling over the situation, ruminating on the reasons for it, feelings of shame and hopelessness cresting in my awareness. It was evening, a vulnerable time for me as it is, and bitterness was clouding my vision. After my daughter went to bed, I launched into my litany of complaints to my husband, who responded with his usual vain attempts to give perspective in the face of my cascade of hopelessness. This elicited my predictable wave of anger at him for minimizing my feelings. I gave him a dirty look and marched upstairs to meditate. Why did I do this? It was really the last thing I wanted to do. However, part of me (my Witness perhaps?) knew that I had made a commitment to myself regarding how I was going to cope with my negativity. I sat down angrily in my little room and began to breathe shallowly and defiantly, as if to say to myself and the universe, "I dare you to get me to feel better." "One, two, three, four, ... " Inhale. Exhale. Breathing growing deeper ... After just a few minutes, I started to lift out of the bitter muck. I peeked at the clock. It had been about ten minutes and I felt quite different. My breathing was obviously deeper. But my thoughts about the situation had also shifted. I felt less oppressed and was able to see myself in action, getting caught in my habitual story line. At that moment, I realized with a great "Aha!" that part of me did not want to feel better. If I were to feel better, then I would have to take full responsibility for the situation—and I didn't want to have to deal with it because of my shame. Somehow, being caught in the litany of my fears and woes, my old story about myself, and thereby living out the shame, was preferable to being a grown-up and coping with the situation directly. If I were to fully accept the situation without shame, then I could take steps to cope directly. "Oh, I see ... this is the meaning of that word 'acceptance' that I'm always using with clients."

Consider how this may apply to your struggle with your weight and food. There is a subjective story line to your experience that is full of your particular pain regarding your relationship to your body. Helplessness and resignation, as I illustrate with my own story, have a magnetic pull in consciousness. And, not to be underestimated, your emotional reactions, particularly that of shame, serve as a powerful nullifier of your personal power. Having a larger body in our society exposes you to ongoing feelings of judgment and rejection. It is the last acceptable prejudice. Shame is poisonous and builds a dark, destructive momentum inside. Without even being aware of it, you can let the assessments of others define you and put parameters on your behavior and define what is and is not possible for you. It is very important for you to ask yourself, "If I could accept the facts of this situation without shame, what would I do about it?" Lifting out of shame empowers you to make self-affirmative choices that embrace possibility rather than act out resignation. You can see with the clear-eyed perspective described by Iyengar—"I have the skills to cope with this situation." The most important aspect of this overall equation is lifting out of the emotional drama, marked by fear, shame, and

helplessness, to a more objective perspective where you can Witness your habitual reactions with intelligence and thereby choose a better course of action.

Frances Kuffel wrote the memoir *Passing for Thin*, which describes with
stunning honesty her experience of losing about two hundred pounds. She
describes her "Aha!" moment after her best friend, who was an alcoholic
himself, had excoriated her for her weight.

> *"'How dare he speak for me and my problems—*
> *he's nothing but a drunk!'*
>
> I can only describe the next moment by saying the ceiling talked back.
> I heard a retort, but not from my brain. It came from outside of myself,
> hovering, watching.
>
> 'And *you are*—?' The ceiling asked me to fill in the blank. I stopped in
> my tracks.
>
> *'I am…'*
> *I am exactly the same.'*
> *'I can't stop eating.'"*

Kuffel goes on to say, "I had no excuses left. Raised on stories of Cath-
erine of Siena and St. Teresa of Avila, I don't ignore talking ceilings. Having read Jung and Shakespeare, I don't ignore the truth."

Interestingly, in Frances's experience, the objective vision that Iyengar
describes is literal—she actually experiences "the truth" emanating from the
ceiling. Her deep insight into herself, the truth of her addiction, comes from
the outside. The ceiling spoke without judgment, and it spoke the truth. This
is how Witnessing works. You'll notice as well that her vision lacks shame. It
is objective. The catalyst to her insight, however, was the shame induced by
her friend's hypocrisy. The pain of this betrayal broke through her denial and
empowered her to take action.

The Witnessing capacity of consciousness does not need to be dramatic, as it was in Frances's case. It can be more subtle daily acknowledgements regarding your behavior, both positive and negative. For example, when you are at a restaurant and wavering between the salad and the cheeseburger, this awareness comes in the simple act of pausing to check in with your gut and realize that you really are not particularly hungry after all and you order the salad. The soft green of the arugula, the crunch of the carrots, and the savory sweetness of the beets are just the thing. You feel nicely satisfied after the meal and you Witness your choice with a nod of acknowledgement. Or conversely, you notice that you are quite hungry and you order a more substantial meal, making sure to round out the meal with a large order of vegetables. And then at another time when you find yourself being irritable with an insurance representative, who is merely the messenger of unwelcome news, you may pause for a moment, check your rudeness, and note your reaction to the in-convenient news. Even when you are Witnessing "bad" behavior in yourself, there can be relief in seeing yourself more objectively and being honest about your strengths and weaknesses. This is similar to how Janice responded to her out-of-control bingeing after she recognized the historical catalyst for her behavior. She realized that the trigger of arbitrary authority awakened a dor-mant rebellious demon inside (a demon she had needed when she was a child and under her father's unpredictable and punitive care). She was able to learn from this experience without punitive self-judgment. If you do find yourself being harsh or judgmental toward yourself, you can Witness this as well, not-ing how pervasive your tendency toward negative self-evaluation is. The im-portant aspect of this is cultivating the ability to see yourself more objectively without becoming swept away by the momentum of the old storyline.

You can enhance your Witnessing capacity by going to psychotherapy or joining a support group, such as a twelve-step program. These venues all allow you to experience feedback from others regarding how they perceive you. However, joining a group can be pretty daunting, especially if you are new to the idea of being Witnessed by others. In that case, individual therapy is generally a safer forum. Journaling is the least threatening way to enhance your Witnessing capacity, though don't underestimate its power. The act of translating your thoughts and feelings into words gives you a different perspective on your experience. Through journaling, you may naturally find yourself problem solving or examining your attitudes and assumptions with more detachment.

Reflections on Your Witness

1. How strong is your Witness? Are you able to step back from situations and objectively assess your responsibility in situations?

2. When you are feeling defensive, what helps you to detach and assess your responsibility in the situation?

3. Consider the role of shame in your relationship to food and your body. Does shame get in the way of Witnessing your behavior honestly and taking more responsibility for change?

4. What activities are you willing to engage in to strengthen your Witness? As mentioned, twelve-step programs, group and individual therapy, and journaling are all tools for this.

Taking Responsibility

Iyengar goes on to discuss how change happens in the personality. Our capacity to objectively Witness ourselves gives way to our ability to then make choices that will bring about new circumstances. In his words, "This first quality [objectivity] makes possible intelligence's second. It can choose. It can choose to perform an action that is new, that is innovative. It can initiate change. It can decide to jump out of the ruts in which we are all stuck and strike out on a path for its own evolution. Intelligence does not chat. It is the quiet, determined, clear-eyed revolutionary of our consciousness." You could say that we have the capacity to harness the power of cause and effect. We harness our intelligence in order to choose new causes as a means to create new effects. The yoga of food is based on this precept because we look beneath the immediate lure of our habits and instead begin to choose based on more objective criteria that is linked to an enhanced appreciation of cause and effect.

In her book *Passing for Thin*, Frances Kuffel's insight into her food addiction (when the ceiling spoke to her) precipitated her engagement with Overeaters Anonymous, and she went on to lose 188 pounds. Talk about revolutionary! Frances is unusual and touching because she has a great capacity to Witness herself and take responsibility for her role in creating her problems. After having major abdominal surgery due to an intestinal blockage, she writes, "Worse, I'd brought it on myself. My intestines were strangled in scarring from the surgery twelve years earlier to remove my gallbladder and a thirty-six-pound ovarian cyst, malfunctioning because of the food I ate and the hormonal imbalances that resulted from my obesity. I was face to face with the most serious consequences of what I had done to my body, had fought for two and a half years to undo, or pretend away." But just because Frances is able to see herself clearly, this does not make her immune to getting derailed by her old habits/samskaras. She has the clarity of objectivity, yet this does not mean that she is able to harness the power of choice consistently. As a sobering aside, it is my understanding is that she fell back under the spell of her food addiction. Two and a half years, the length of time it took Frances to lose weight, is not long at all compared to a lifetime of abusing food. This illustrates the point that Alcoholics Anonymous often makes—the only thing that stands between a person with twenty years of recovery and a full relapse is one little drink. In yoga language, you might say, "Don't underestimate your samskaras!" The importance of moving slowly and deliberately is paramount. Respect the enormity of your work and the power of your shame, despair, and habitual patterns to cajole, deceive, and entrap you with their false promises of relief. Keep in mind too that you will have to face consequences from your past behavior, and you can't undo this quickly. As Frances indicated above, you can't "pretend away" the consequences of your past behavior. If you, like Frances, have lived life buffered by food and a haze of serial carbo-highs, you too may feel walloped by life without the protection that food addiction and extra weight confer. Being a revolutionary in your own life means staying focused on the small gestures that bring sanity to your day-to-day life and honing your ability to be present to all of your feelings, no matter how bleak and despairing they may be. This means being firm and compassionate with your tendency to self-sabotage. Self-sabotage is a term that refers to the ubiquitous tendency to resign ourselves to the status quo, the rut of our old identity, and ignore the power of choice and re-creation that is always present. We all do it. It is comfortable. It is boring. And we all, always, have the option to not do it. That is scary. That is exciting. That is revolutionary!

Iyengar himself uses food to illustrate the importance of the little choices we face every day regarding how we care for ourselves. "Time pauses in a moment of awareness and reflection in which suddenly our destiny is ours to command. 'Do I eat a second scoop of ice cream or do I stop now?' The choice may be hard, but at least it is simple. We find ourselves at a parting of the ways that, however trivial in itself, is somehow momentous to us."

Let me repeat his words: "The choice may be hard, but at least it is simple." Isn't that the crux of the matter? One of my clients once said to me in a moment of great frustration over her out-of-control eating—"It's not like it's rocket science!" Well, no. Perhaps rocket science would be easier for us to master than the momentary whims and deeper longings of our physical/ emotional bodies. I find it interesting that Iyengar includes such a phrase, "our destiny is ours to command," in a discussion about ice cream. These moments may seem trivial and yet they are, as he points out, momentous. If you step back from the situation, if you Witness the string of seemingly discrete decisions about what to put in your body and when, you can see that being able to take a stand during these small, invisible moments signifies your willingness to steer your own ship with intelligence. This says a great deal about your approach to your life. The enormity of our human ability to make choices is astounding. We really can be revolutionaries in our own lives if we are willing to utilize the power of the Witness and make intelligent choices, however small they may be at the time. According to Iyengar, "This is history being made, your personal history, thanks to the mirror and scissors of intelligence—see, choose, act."

The yoga of food harnesses the **above credo—"see, choose, act."** You step back and see your habits without excuses or explanations—and without shame! You harness your ability to choose, which immediately opens up new vistas of possibilities. You act on these new choices. New things then become possible. Your choices need not be grand or momentous. In fact, they may be quite humble. You take a walk, cook a vegetable, take a deep breath, attend a yoga class. When the consequences of past behaviors rear their ugly head, you nod and say hello, but keep your eyes on the path in front of you. Easier said than done. And of course you will at times look back and feel regret, shame, or despair. But you also remember that these are just feelings, and the power of new choice and action is always present. Cultivating this awareness is a skill and an ability that we all have. It just takes practice, patience, and heart. And we all have those capacities as well.

Reflections on Responsibility and Your Health

1. How willing are you to take responsibility for your choices in your life? Are you one of those people who is overly responsible for others but not able to take full responsibility for yourself?

2. Do you have rescue fantasies? The handsome prince, or the new pill, that will somehow relieve you of the burden of choice and action?

3. What are some small, concrete ways that you could take more responsibility for your health today?

Your Issues Are in Your Tissues

In our society, we often tend to ignore what our bodies are telling us and instead are encouraged to medicate the symptoms with sleeping pills, stool softeners, a few beers, and a burrito. The problem with this approach is that whatever your body is trying to tell you gets lost beneath your attempts to cover it up. The problem goes deeper and manifests in more and more pernicious ways. Tapping into your larger intelligence, the Witness, involves opening to the messages held in your cellular body. In Iyengar's words, "To gain health, you have to know the unconscious mind, which expresses itself within the nervous system." When you are in a subjective mode, which means you are caught up in your habitual story line, you have a problem (you can't sleep, you are overweight, anxious, whatever), you don't like it (Clever-mind/manas says, "Problem bad. Fix it!"), you seek the solution—and in our pill popping, purse-peddling society, you will surely find one offered. So you obscure the problem with a pill, a purse, a new car, or a new workout plan. Whatever your body was expressing is now underground, covered over by the distraction of your "solution." This is a lost opportunity to learn from your nervous system because your symptom is now latent. You are unable to Witness, and thereby respond meaningfully to, the message held in the tissues of your body.

In order to gain access to the unconscious mind through your body, as Iyengar suggests, you must be able to set aside the attraction/aversion reflex of your Clever-mind/manas and the attachments of your Egoic-self/ahamkara. Clever-mind/manas is invested in quick solutions to problems, while your Egoic-self/ahamkara is attached to particular views about yourself, either positive ("I'm a healthy person") or negative (I'm fat"). Getting to know your body is a process that requires openness and humility, which are qualities of the Witness. Your Egoic-self/ahamkara won't like everything that you find. Perhaps you will discover, as I did, that you are not as "healthy" as you wanted to believe. You will need to experience living in (integrate the unfolding of) your body in a way that allows for the inconsistencies and disappointments inherent to real life in a real body. You will be forced to face damage, effects secondary to cause (that's karma), wrought from your prior habits. In the words of Frances Kuffel, "My belly looked like Normandy from twenty thousand feet, hedgerows, canals, craters, and one big highway right through my navel." It is not an accident that she uses a war metaphor to describe the signs of carnage on her flesh. In our society, we often battle ourselves every day— some fad diets even call it "the battle of the bulge"—so thinking of the body as war zone is not unusual. And healing from the damages incurred requires us to concede whatever projections of perfection and completion that we have associated with getting "thin" or "healthy." Instead we commit to facing the damages with compassion and resoluteness regarding our intention to heal. This requires great heart as we come to terms with the damages left behind from the various wars being waged on the ground of our flesh. Sophie, who had lost 100 pounds, told me that the reason she is not swimming yet, and a large part of what led to her start regaining her weight, was the realization that the excess skin on her body was not going anywhere regardless of her efforts in the gym or further weight loss. She was profoundly disappointed that her Herculean effort to reshape her body, though successful, left remnants from her past that could not be erased by the prodigious powers of will alone. The shame and disappointment that she felt threatened to catapult her back smack into the middle of her addiction. And here, she showed the most Herculean effort of all—she decided to get help through therapy. She lifted out of her shame and chose another way.

After her hysterectomy, Cindy was painfully fixated on the things that she perceived were still wrong with her body. Yes, her pelvic pain was greatly reduced. But she was still suffering from ongoing ailments, aches, pains, and other indignities that irritated her and diluted her sense of success about the surgery. "I don't want to accept that these things are still wrong," she stated, as if her refusal to accept would change the conditions in her body. I think we can all relate to this stance, unproductive as it may be. We don't like how something is and we cling to this aversion and act as if whatever it is we don't like doesn't exist. If you have ever run up credit card debt, overeaten to the point of discomfort, drank too much alcohol, or gone over the speed limit, then you know what I am talking about. Cindy tended to take this position in many areas of her life and used her precious energy to lament choices she has made or not made, as if regret could somehow magically undo the past. Like her body, her life has circumstances that she feels, from her subjective perspective, cannot be remedied. As long as this is where her attention is fixated, this is where her attention will stay, and her perception of futility will remain true. The aches, pains, and imperfections of her body and her life will capture her gaze and obliterate the concomitant rightness and possibility inherent within both. The possibility for change, the different choices that lie immediately before her, are invisible to the subjective eye caught in the story line of complaint and misery.

Stepping away and glimpsing the whirlpool of complaint (the samskara/ habit) sounds so easy. As a therapist, sitting in my chair, the different possibilities that lay before someone else are plain to see. Yet, who doesn't get caught up in hopelessness and futility, flailing for some ground in the midst of untoward events, primal fears, and petty mishaps? Building a habit of self-reflection and cultivating a space where the Witness can grow will help you to find some ground amidst it all. The ground you immediately find is your body, your breath, and your heartbeat. With all of its imperfections, your body provides a resting place for your weary, pleasure-seeking, nitpicking, stubborn, yet oh so Clever-mind. And it is here, in this resting place of your body, in this space of the small yet eternal present moment, wherein lies the embryo of change.

For all of us, change begins with coaxing engagement in the here and now circumstances of our lives in small, simple ways that lift us out of the preoccupation with damages we deem too far gone for human intervention. For Cindy, these activities include cooking, walking, and brief daily meditations. Sophie is similar to Cindy in that she can waste energy lamenting conditions in her body that feel unfixable. For her, change involves a one-day-at-a-time attitude and giving herself permission to focus on her well-being beneath the skin. She is curtailing obsessive exercise, journaling her feelings, and focusing on healing relationships with her family. She has also started swimming again and is finding great pleasure in reengaging with this sensual, playful activity from her childhood. For both women, the change process starts with finding and repeating small commitments that can build upon themselves. These simple engagements in the present moment, starting with breathing more fully, make room for the body to come alive. You are no longer engaged in running from, covering over, or arguing with what your body is saying, but rather cultivating a space of openness wherein you can begin to learn from your tissues.

No matter what symptoms you may or may not have, your attitude toward your body will be manifested in your health. If you have a contentious, hateful, or impatient attitude toward your flesh, you will suffer. Many of my clients struggle with overt self-hatred. Kimberly, a devoted twelve-stepper who determinedly addresses her "stuff" with her sponsor and with me, hates her stomach. She shivers with disgust when we talk about "it." She also can't stand her mother, whom she refers to as Paula, her first name. Kimberly describes her mother as a passive-aggressive, guilting, and cloying figure. An example that rings out from her childhood is when her mother had stomach surgery. Kimberly was twelve years old and recalls her mother repeatedly showing her the sutures in her stomach and laughing patronizingly at Kimberly's horrified response. Isn't it interesting that now as an adult Kimberly struggles with hatred for her own stomach? We have explored these issues lodged in her tissues several times in therapy and I wish that I could say that she now loves and accepts herself fully, including the offensive flesh comprising her belly. Not quite. Though she did share with me recently that her husband had commented that he liked the softness of her body, including her stomach, and this appeared to soften her harshness toward herself. Perhaps love does heal all. And perhaps her work in therapy and the twelve steps has opened her enough to be able to receive her husband's affirmation of all of her. Something that her mother was unable to do.

Reflections on What Your Body Is Telling You

1. Choose a physical issue—it can be anything, an ache or pain, your stomach, your breasts, indigestion, chronic headaches. Sit down with your journal and start a dialogue between yourself and your symptom. It might go like this:

   Self: "Why the hell are you so damn big? I feel ashamed of you and am sick of having to cover you up all the time."

   Belly: "It really hurts me when you talk to me that way. It makes me churn and tighten into a little ball."

   Self: "Oh, yeah. I wish you would turn into a little ball. Then I wouldn't be so embarrassed."

   Belly: "Maybe if you were a little nicer to me we could work together."

   Self: "Hmmm...what do you mean?"

   Belly: "I'm dying here. I feel so ashamed the way you treat me. It makes me sick! It reminds me of how the kids used to laugh at me in phys ed. It makes me just want to give up!"

   Self: "Oh...I think I'm beginning to get it."

   This is just an example. Find your own voice here and let your imagination guide you. This exercise can actually be kind of fun as you create a voice for your physical body. Ask questions like "What do you need from me?" or "What are you trying to tell me?" as a way to open up the dialogue.

2. Do you struggle with an uncomfortable physical issue? What is your approach to this issue? Are you avoidant? Are there things you could and should do to address it? What stops you from doing this? Might you feel relieved if you take the ball and do what you need to do before it gets worse?

Creating a Pause

Creating a pause between impulse and action is how you begin to intervene at the level of your samskaras. So many of our choices are knee-jerk, habitual reactions. We rarely pause to think about the wisdom of our choices, especially if we have had certain patterns for years. If this is just, "who I am" or "how I do things," then you are trapped within that story line. Creating space allows the pause wherein your Witness can have an "Aha!" moment that will allow something different in your life to unfold. You step out of the subjective story line, reassess your complaints, and take stock of your responsibility for the situation. Then, with the clear-eyed vision that Iyengar described earlier, you consider the things that you can do about it. Your Witness has stepped in to intervene between cause and effect. In his words, "It is the momentary pause in the process of cause and effect that allows us to begin the process of freedom."

I am going to illustrate how this works with a seemingly trivial example from my own life in a body. Recently, I woke up after having attended a party the night before, feeling very uncomfortable in my body. My stomach was bloated and my appetite was blunted. I was somewhat affronted by this turn of events because I had thought I was very restrained in my consumption at the party (Egoic-self/ahamkara says, "Who me? Overeat? Not!"). I also have this odd reaction to feeling overfull, which is an intensification of wanting to eat. Since at a deep level food is my "go to" in order to feel better, that's what my Clever-mind/manas wants. Due to my longtime positive habit/samskara of exercise, I refrained from this tendency and instead took my bilious body out for an extended cycling venture. About twenty minutes after lacing up my shoes, my body, taking on the rhythm of movement and my mind loosening from its rut of affront and complaint, I recognized that yes, in spite of restraining myself the night before, I had indeed overindulged. There was no shame in my recognition, just the nod of "Yes, there you are again." It was no longer a big deal, and I considered steps I could take to remedy my discomfort.

In this example, my exercise routine created a pause between cause and effect. So, rather than stew in the unpleasantness of a bloated body that was paradoxically wanting some hair of the dog to medicate the discomfort, I opened up some space that allowed me to feel better, accept my responsibility for the situation, and assess ways that I could cope with it realistically.

You'll notice in this little scenario that initially I was arguing with my body. My body was saying, "You ate too much." My Egoic-self was saying, "Get out! I did not." If my Egoic-self was to have her way, she would continue to eat just to show that damn body that it wasn't true. And then, following this cascade of events, the volume of complaint would be turned way up, drowning out any hope of taking meaningful action to feel better. In order to open up space for the Witness, and to find the intelligence to do this, you must have some tools so that you don't resort to the "stuff" you normally fill that space with. The "stuff" may be food, alcohol, pills, gossip, complaining, shoes, drama… Your tools may be journaling, walking, yoga or aerobic exercise, or meditation.

Sometimes merely changing your routine can create a pause and open up space for the Witness. Janice, for example, decided to give up drive-thrus for Lent. She described for me the intoxicating anonymity created by the drive-thru experience. In the privacy of her car, she could order whatever she wanted in whatever quantity she desired and not have to endure the judgment of others or be accountable for her behavior. "You don't even have to see their faces when they hand you the food. All you can see are their shoulders and arms." I visualized disembodied arms handing over grease-stained bags, the description evoking that of an illicit drug deal or sexual encounter.

During her period of abstinence from drive-thrus, she and a friend went to Taco Bell. Janice, true to her commitment, held firm even in the face of her friend's offer to go into the restaurant for her. No, Janice knew that she needed to be accountable for the food, so she went inside the restaurant and ordered food for both of them. Her friend had declined a soda so there was only one drink, which made it look like all the food was for her. "I had to order the food and then stand there and wait for it. It was so uncomfortable," she later recounted to me, writhing in the leftover discomfort, but also with a look of pride on her face. We agreed that it was really good for her to face her fears of judgment and to be more accountable internally for what she was putting into her body. Refraining from the pattern of anonymous consumption created a pause, wherein she was able to take more responsibility for her behavior. Although this was uncomfortable, it was also refreshing as it lifted her out of the stale habit/samskara of her addiction. She is considering continuing this commitment even after Lent is over.

Reflections on Your Space

1. Do you have ritual pauses in your day? These are times when you are not doing, fulfilling, obsessing, planning, or eating. Prayer, meditation, journaling all create a pause. TV and reading do not, as they distract from, rather than open up, your interior experience.

2. Do you have compulsive behaviors, such as Janice's, that create pain in your life? Do you dare to interrupt this pattern so as to create some space to Witness yourself?

3. What is the "stuff" that you are most likely to fill empty space with? What tools/habits would you like to cultivate that will instead help you to open up space?

How Therapy Can Help

Therapy can have multiple functions in your life. It can create a space between cause and effect, wherein you allow yourself to be witnessed by another. As you act out your issues with your therapist, which I will illustrate, your therapist can mirror them back to you in a respectful, compassionate way. If you feel safe enough to stay open to this, you will begin to see how you repeat the same patterns in virtually all areas of your life, including with your body and your food. At other times, your therapist can function as a sounding board who directs you inward to discover your own wisdom. Ultimately, therapy serves as a useful tool in your quest to develop more insight and Witnessing capacity into your deeper, often hidden, tendencies.

Cindy had an idealizing transference with me. An idealizing transference refers to a client's need to see the therapist as "perfect." Cindy saw me as the perfect yogini, calm and centered, picking tea leaves in my back yard. "But you're thin!" she once practically accused, as if that conferred some kind of superhuman status.

Cindy's wish that I was perfect was indicative of her idealized fantasies about herself and the hidden belief or hope that someday, somehow she would find her "perfect" self. We discussed her unrealistic view of me and what this said about her—her need to have someone perfect show her the way and how this would help her attain some idealized status in her own life. Her idealized feelings, however, didn't budge and she seemed disbelieving that I was actually real. The one-dimensional image she had of me mirrored her relationship with herself. If I was "thin," need-less, and satisfied, then she was "fat," needy, and unsatisfied. Perhaps through osmosis, or a diet, she could obtain what she projected that I had—a life without struggle, deprivation, or shame.

A near crisis occurred in our relationship when I was having difficulty receiving payment from her insurance because I didn't get proper authorization for multiple sessions. We were both triggered: she was triggered due to fears that she would be charged for my error; I was triggered by my fear that

I was not going to be reimbursed for hours of work. It was important for Cindy to experience me as imperfect, but also as not retaliating against her for her disappointment in me. I had to work with myself not to be defensive about my error or blaming of her for the predicament we were in. Thankfully, we were both able to use this incident effectively to help her integrate my lack of perfection, yet still maintain our relationship wherein she was able to still see me in a generally positive light. "I realize your job is more than sitting in a comfortable chair," she said to me not long after this.

The next incident occurred perhaps eight months later when she expressed frustration about our work together. We unpacked this and she was able to express feeling disappointed that I had not directed her more firmly in the treatment. She revealed seeing my "weakness" as a therapist and said at other times she was very aware of my sadness. This was a pivotal moment in the therapy in that she palpably experienced my realness, my lack of perfection, and was again able to express her frustration to me directly. In turn, she experienced me responding to her feedback openly and shifting my approach so as to meet her needs more effectively. I took care to be more structured during our sessions so as to meet her need for more direction. It also allowed us to talk about her other relationships, which she tends to cut off as soon as she is disappointed. The fact that she was able to express her disappointment in me directly, rather than cutting off, was a new, healing experience for her. We discussed how in the past, ambivalence has dominated her approach to others and to herself. Ambivalence literally means *ambi*—"two," *valence*—"directions." Ambivalence, thus, is going in two directions at the same time, as in "I love it. I hate it." This is not a very effective use of energy! Think of how you may live this dynamic out with food, your body, and perhaps other areas of your life. Cindy lived this out with herself ("I'm great!" oscillating with "I'm a failure!"), as well as in her relationships with her family of origin and her husband. Our work in therapy gave her a new experience of integration with me, which will later allow her to integrate her own "weakness" and sadness. It will also eventually help her to better manage her relationship with food—"I want it. I shouldn't have it." or "I hate it. I love it." can be replaced with "Is this good for me?" Or "Does this serve my greater well-being?"

My clients often ask me for advice during sessions. Sometimes I will give direct advice, but more often than not I will probe for my clients' own answer. This is not merely hedging on my part. Rather, it is in response to the common human tendency to defer, to look to another for direction and ignore one's own internal compass. My job as a therapist is to first help a client identify and then polish his or her own internal compass regarding what he or she feels or needs and what direction needs to be taken to meet these needs. Hopefully, you can see how this translates to the dinner table. It's the need to look at a book, diet plan, or other person regarding what and how to eat versus looking inside and making decisions based upon your own needs and constitution. The yoga of food prioritizes your ability to choose what works for you.

The other day, Janice brought up an interesting question. She finds it helpful to compartmentalize herself into a parent-child dyad. Her parent-self exhibits the kind, rational intelligence that she is quite capable of exerting when she is not emotionally triggered. Her child-self is the ravenous, angry energy that takes over when she is triggered or even just eating rich food and wanting more. "Should I imagine myself as an abusive parent who is going to parenting class to become a better parent or should I imagine myself as a loving parent who has inherited an abused child?" As we talked it through, I probed about how she would parent a ravenous, angry child. Janice discussed ways she would provide limits with warmth, firmness with understanding. She knows that although she rebels with outrage at arbitrary authority, she actually longs for sane, stable structure in her own life. This provides a good example of how therapy works: Janice was not asking me what to do or how to feel, but instead was using therapy as an opportunity to think out loud and talk through her interior experience. At the end of the session, Janice asked, "Is it really strange that I think this way about myself?" She was referring to her creation of an internal parent-child split. I replied, "If it works for you and helps you better understand yourself, then go with it!" There is a great feeling of freedom, perhaps even revelry, as you uncover and indulge your own grand uniqueness and quirkiness. If others may consider this strange or unconventional, so be it. As you grow more comfortable with your special brand of uniqueness, you bring this freedom to the dinner table where you also indulge your knowledge of what works for you and your body. If others think you are strange, overeating or undereating, so be it. There is freedom in daring to be yourself and therapy can and should encourage full ownership of your unique self.

Reflections on Participating in Therapy

1. Have you ever been in therapy? What are your biases or preconceived notions about it?

2. Consider how therapy might be a tool for you in your quest for greater health and well-being. Think about what it would be like for you to share your issues with food and your body with another person.

Yoga Practice as a Mirror

"How you do one thing is how you do everything," Diana, the beautiful, sensual teacher from my neighborhood studio intones suggestively as she leads us through the morning vinyasa. Then she snorts with laughter. We all know what she's talking about. When you consistently practice yoga, your mat becomes a personal laboratory where you study your approach to life, to work, rest, sex, food, and to being in a body. You cultivate objectivity and curiosity about your patterns and get interested in how you've taken up this brief opportunity to be incarnated on this troubled, beautiful planet of ours. Even if you find that your approach to your life is haphazard, clumsy, lacking in sensuality or grace, that's okay. The point is to begin looking, observing, noting without judgment and noting your judgment as well. Hence, your yoga practice becomes a place to Witness your approach to work and to rest. To beginnings and endings, pleasure and pain. Iyengar puts it this way: "What is the advantage conferred by the mirror of intelligence? Simply that we can see ourselves as if from a distance. Suddenly the Egoic-self becomes an object. Normally it is the subject, incapable of seeing things except from its own point of view."

Through my yoga practice, I have become acutely aware that I often dread and avoid beginning focused work. Witnessing my procrastination allows me to work with this habit by approaching difficult tasks in a more no-nonsense kind of way. "Now, Melissa," I say to myself, "don't fritter away your time. Get to it!" Change is made possible by observing your patterns and then, when you are ready, making an effort to shift out of your habitual pattern/ samskara. But it can't be a top-down change, as in "You'd better change this problem now!" This is punitive and controlling and it doesn't work because it reinforces shame. There must be time given to containing and allowing the self that you are to just Be as you look on and observe yourself from the side. Your self-observation during your yoga practice will at first consist of inchoate whispers regarding your patterns. You may notice yourself comparing your practice to the person next to you and competing with her so as to do it better. One day, as you are doing this, the teacher's words may penetrate, "This is not a competition." Or "How you do one thing is how you do everything," and it suddenly strikes you how absurd your thoughts are. You realize how you do the same comparisons at your office and with your friends. This is an "Aha!" moment when your Witness quietly smiles with the pleasure of self-recognition. There is no shame in your recognition; rather, you experience a deeper understanding of what it means to be human. You also realize that the more you can know these patterns, the less controlled you are by them, and the more you understand others as well.

Yoga provides a mirror to learn about how you cope with both pleasure and pain. If you want to learn more about how you react to pain, you start by creating your own strife deliberately so that you can deal with the inevitable pain that will greet you on your path through life. In Iyengar's words, "Back bends, for example, allow us to see the courage and tenacity of people, to see whether they can bear the pain." I usually dread my back-bend series. I have Witnessed that my sequence of back bends takes me an inordinately long time to complete. This is due to me lying down and daydreaming between the poses. My flaccidity of mind and body is a metaphor for how I often fritter away time in the rest of my life. And it causes stress because after wasting time, I am then running late and not able to enjoy free and clear relaxation, let alone the enjoyment of giving myself over more fully to my work. This realization has helped me manage my time better during my practice. I set a timer and am firmer with myself about not resting too long. But as I said above, I aim to not do this with a punitive tone toward myself, but rather because I understand that it is for my own benefit.

Pleasure is also a part of life and a part of yoga practice. You likely give priority to one side of the pleasure-pain polarity, which is indicative of your style of navigating life's inevitable ups and downs. Relaxation and work need to be in balance in your life and there is a high likelihood that you emphasize one over the other. Though I don't consider myself a masochist, I do tend to emphasize pain over pleasure. I "get things over with" (pain) so I can get to some reward on the other side (pleasure). Pleasure must be earned and it comes in regimented doses, often in the form of food. Through my yoga practice, the dichotomous way I was structuring things became clearer and clearer to me, "Get the yoga practice over with so I can have a meal." Slowly, through consistent practice, I began to notice the exquisite pleasure wrought from the practice itself. Rather than something to "get through," it could be something to savor. For example, holding a difficult pose and then releasing it creates a rush of warmth and well-being that feels really good. Deep forward bends are very relaxing, especially when placed toward the end of a class. Any pose where your head is hanging down feels soothing, as does stretching your head back and opening your throat in back bends. So, rather than yoga practice being something to get through, I began to notice how the interplay between pleasure (relaxation) and pain (effort) constitute the heart of the practice.

Noticing your relationship to pleasure and pain in your yoga practice provides insight into your relationship with food. Interestingly, many women with food issues will admit that deep down, they don't really enjoy food or eating all that much. Think of Janice, who told me, "I use my body as a garbage disposal." That image certainly doesn't evoke pleasure! Then there's Mandy, who wants to write a book called "How I Learned to Hate the Food I Love." Any compulsion negates pleasure. Reclaiming your capacity for pleasure away from the dinner table (away from your compulsive trigger) is essential to reclaiming pleasure in food. Many experts on food disorders will tell you just to sit down and enjoy your food. Sounds so simple, doesn't it? I think, however, that in order to do this you first have to build insight into your patterns of tension and rigidity in your body, and in your life, before you can do something so natural as enjoying a meal. The patterns of tension and rigidity are firmly entrenched in your mind and body and will be most active when you are around food if you have struggled with your relationship to food. Discovering what it feels like to relax or feel good in your body away from food will help you to recover feelings of well-being while eating food. This will take time due to possibly having spent years feeling shame or ambivalence around your need to eat and the pleasure of eating. Sophie provides a good example of this, who, as I previously mentioned, looked somewhat bashful when she "admitted" to liking yogurt with granola. In order to claim her right to this pleasure, she must also claim her right to pleasure away from the dinner table. For now, she is able to safely experience some sensual pleasure in the shower and while swimming. The seeds of pleasure will germinate here and as she grows more comfortable, will allow her to discover other avenues for this essential human need and birthright.

My own history of body-shame still provides a backdrop to my experience of food. I vividly remember sitting at the round wooden dinner table in the echoey dining hall at boarding school. I was fifteen or so and deep into my compulsive-eating disorder. The young girl next to me suggests, contempt not veiled beneath her guise of helpfulness, "You really should eat more vegetables." Then there was the scathing contempt from a male acquaintance who had not seen me for twenty or thirty pounds, "Fat girls don't have any fun, you know," he informed me imperiously. For some reason, when you are overweight, people feel that they can treat you like you're an idiot. These experiences of humiliation lay down tracks in the nervous system (think deep grooves/samskaras). And now you're just supposed to sit down and enjoy a meal? No, pleasure must be rediscovered away from the dinner plate and what better place than the yoga mat? You'll notice here, as I quote particularly searing comments from my personal experience that I am sharing with you my conditioning. These past events have much less power over me now because I have pulled these memories out of the sea of preconscious memory and shone the light of awareness upon them. These comments resonate from the past and are not particularly relevant to my life now. The tracks are still there in my nervous system, however, which means I remain vulnerable to judgment about my body from others. Knowing this about myself allows me to more easily identify the shame when this occurs and Witness my habitual response to judgment before getting caught up in an unproductive, reactive response.

Reflections on Your Internal Experience

1. When you practice yoga, be attentive to the stream of thoughts and feelings that you have during the experience. You may notice dread, fear, accomplishment, comparisons, etc. Consider whether this stream of thoughts accompany you during other daily endeavors.

2. Jot down what you learn about yourself in a journal. Be careful of your tendency to criticize yourself when you find traits in yourself that you don't care for. Work with the idea of accepting yourself, right here and now, just the way you are.

3. What is the ratio of pleasure and pain in your life? Which side of the polarity do you favor? Are you more fearful of pleasure or pain?

4. What are your non-food sources of pleasure? How often do you experience these?

Your Inner Guru

When you come across a particularly charismatic, gifted, or attractive yoga teacher, you may find yourself developing an idealizing transference with him or her. As described above, an idealizing transference occurs when you project unrealistic fantasies onto another person. Yoga teachers provide lightning rods for this tendency because they are often very attractive and very fit. It is easy to imagine that they are perfect human specimens and to project unrealistic fantasies onto them. The danger with this is that if you aren't aware of this tendency in yourself, you may begin to emulate this person in a way that blocks the development of your own intuition about what is right for you. If your yoga teacher is vegan, well then, maybe you should be vegan too. And that tattoo on her lower back looks really cool. And where does she buy those hot yoga clothes?

Iyengar addresses the pitfalls of this tendency as well. "I sometimes tell my pupils that the practice they do in yoga class is not, strictly speaking, yoga practice. The reason for this is that in a class, although you are undoubtedly 'doing' and, hopefully, learning you are subordinate to a teacher. The directing intelligence comes from him, and you follow to the best of your ability. At home, on the other hand, it is your own intelligence that is the master, and the progress that you make is yours and will be maintained. In addition, the will that you employ is yours. It is not derived from the power, the charisma, the strength, or the fieriness of the teacher."

Learning to trust and honor your own wisdom is vital to sustained personal growth. Real confidence comes from trusting your intuition and trusting yourself to listen to it. You may have no idea what is right for you, what to eat, how much to eat, or when to eat. And that's just the food! How about what to do with your life, how to spend your time, and whom to marry? You must slow down the train! When I was a beginning therapy student, I was instructed to allow clients to sit in their confusion. This was a tall order for me because I was already stewing in my own confusion about myself, whether I could ever learn to do therapy, what I should say, what I should wear, never mind what to have for dinner. Sitting with another's confusion felt virtually impossible, especially when they were looking to me for answers. But really, this was quite wise advice from my teachers because it is in this space of confusion, the gap between cause and effect, that you learn to look and feel into what is right for you. I needed to allow clients to find themselves in this space. So, too, in your own life. You must be able to allow yourself to make mistakes in this process of learning to trust yourself. An experimental attitude is best—"I'll try this and see if it works for me." This requires a flexible attitude with yourself, a willingness to admit you don't know everything, and willingness to make mistakes along the way.

I had a dream that I should cut down on coffee. The message came from an old supervisor who showed up during the night and delivered this simple suggestion. I had been having significant digestive issues at the time that were giving me a great deal of distress. Clever-mind/manas says, "Discomfort bad." So I was searching out cures in the form of different supplements, cutting out gluten, this, that, and the other thing. Nothing was working. Then this dream came. "What the . . . ?" My logical mind said, "What could coffee have to do with my problem?" After all, coffee does have antioxidants, right? And even Iyengar mentions having a cup of coffee in his book. If it's good enough for him, then it's good enough for me, I rationalized to myself. So I ignored the dream for several months. Mind you, I don't have a light addiction to coffee. I have been imbibing coffee since the womb. Supposedly, my mother drank pots of coffee during her pregnancy with me.

Then I was off the stuff for fifteen years, other than a warm, milky, sugary cup my parents would allow me now and then.

When I was verging on fifteen and went to boarding school, I re-found coffee. It eased the trauma of leaving my mother at such a young age. Besides, the school had a room devoted to the stuff. A large, industrial coffee pot filled with a nasty brew was the centerpiece of the dilapidated old building with a vomit-stained couch in the corner. Somehow, it represented comfort. Yes, it tasted bad, but I was determined to conquer this minor inconvenience in the service of elbowing my way into the big league of cynical, unafraid adolescents around me. Having watched my mother dreamily consume coffee over the years, I decided that my time had come. At a deep level, it was a substitute for her and I drank it copiously. For me, coffee was linked with achievement, energy, and getting things done. It had no calories, pumped you up for action, and had a laxative and diuretic effect to boot (both perks in my book). Over the years, I drank it whenever. Nothing better than going to an evening class, sixteen ounces in hand, ready for action. Feeling bored? Tired in the afternoon? It was my solution to all my troubles, my consolation prize, I suppose. I didn't stop to notice how it made me feel.

Fast forward to my forties. By this time, post-pregnancy and breastfeeding, during which I had managed to cut down significantly, my morning dose had crept back to its former revered status. I remember early in treatment with my naturopath she had tentatively suggested that I stop coffee. The door snapped shut in my eyes and she had the wisdom to discreetly change direction. "Back away from the pose, sister, or you might get hurt." Now, here I was blatantly ignoring a clear gift from my unconscious mind. So hooked into the addiction, no pause between cause and effect, continuing to live out my habit/samskara. I tell you this to illustrate how pig-headed one can be when comfort ("This is the way I do things") is at stake. I also recount this tale to illustrate that if you are willing to slow down and, well, smell the coffee, you begin to find the answers inside of yourself.

With regard to Iyengar's words above, feel out what is right for you. Try some yoga classes with different teachers and styles. Try some yoga DVDs, again experimenting with different teachers and styles. And practice some on your own if it moves you. The beauty of your meditation is that unless you are in a meditation group, which would likely only convene once a week anyway, you are very much on your own. This may be difficult for you if you don't like your own company. I encourage you to stay with the practice regardless. Sitting initially just for five or ten minutes a day is a first step to opening the door and getting more comfortable with your own confusion and pigheadedness. Over time, comfort with your confusion will allow you to feel into and access your latent intelligence.

With regard to the yoga of food, it is important to access your inner intelligence regarding what foods and what amounts work for you. There is so much nutritional information in our media, and if you haven't noticed, much of it is contradictory. There is an almost religious zeal about the competing information—the paleo-camp versus the vegans is almost as polarized as Christians versus atheists. You must look inside and commit to learning from your own body and be mindful of your tendency to identify with an external, moralistic view that may obliterate your natural body-intelligence. Certainly do your research regarding the benefits of different eating styles, but make sure that it is balanced with internal exploration of your own body-intuition.

As with all things in life, there is a balance between the need for others and the need to look inward. If you are too solipsistic and do not allow yourself to learn from others, then you can become isolated and closed off from your blind spots. Conversely, if you are overly eager for guidance and easily swayed by others, you lose out on developing your own wisdom and intuition about what is right for you. You need balance between containing your experience internally and sharing your experience with others. The windows must be open in your consciousness to allow information in, and you must be able to contain this information so as to use it for your benefit.

Reflections on the Guru in You

1. Do you tend to look outward to others for guidance on how you should do things, or are you more isolated and closed off from others?

2. Do you pay attention to your dreams?

3. Do you trust your intuition about the big things in your life? How about the small things? If you don't, what are your thoughts about how to repair your inward trust?

4. Are you prone to idealizing others? Or do you disparage others and tend to be more judgmental and cynical? You may find that you do both.

5. Some people find their own company difficult to tolerate. Does this apply to you? Or, conversely, do you shy away from relationships with others? Whichever side of the polarity you lean toward, are you willing to push the envelope of your comfort level? How will this benefit you?

Re-Minding Yourself as a Daily Practice

Anna is a tall, angular older woman with startling blue eyes and thick white hair. Her accent is a rich brogue, reflecting her early roots in Scotland. Anna has struggled with a searing depression her entire adult life. She survived a serious suicide attempt in her early twenties, which she has never repeated. However, she describes having had long, dark periods in her life during which she has felt utterly barren internally. A dutiful wife and mother, she would cook food for her family that nauseated her due to her gnarled emotional state. For Anna, food is often a chore and when she is not emotionally well, she has to force herself to eat. Her relationship to food reflects her difficulty taking in and enjoying the small pleasures that life has to offer.

Now in her early seventies, Anna is better than she has ever been. She has learned to relax in bed with a book and deeply wants to enjoy all the gifts life has to offer. She has developed a yoga and meditation practice and is receptive to learning more about herself in this contemplative way. Her depressions are no longer as severe or as long as they were in her earlier days. She is fully aware of how the stark environment in which she was reared seeped into her bones and she knows that now her work involves continually re-minding herself of the goodness that life has to offer. Our sessions are spaced several weeks apart. During this time, she often "forgets" to do the things that inspire her and give her a sense of hope and meaning. We speak of books and ideas that she has found inspiring, like the Buddhist mitri prayer or Pema Chödrön's writing, and she will say, "Oh my, yes. I don't know why I haven't thought to do that." Or "Yes, I must pick up her book again."

Anna does not forget because she is not serious or committed to her growth. She "forgets" because she gets caught in the sweep of her habitual pattern of depression. Our childhood conditioning creates the default setting for how we ordinarily live our lives. The discipline required is finding daily rituals of self-care that re-mind you of the larger scope of what life has to offer and what it possible for you. For Anna, meditation can reinforce the barrenness of her inner world. She describes her practice as being flat and lifeless at times. This is not because this is just how she is or who she is. Rather, it is because this is a state of being that she is prone to. Knowing this about herself, Anna can consciously seek out methods to remember the pleasures life has to offer. She needs a basket of tools that bring color and warmth into her surroundings and her interior world and she needs to have this basket beside her in a very visible way in her life. We plan for her to write of list of intentions in the evening that outline two or three things she will do the next day that lift her up. Listening to music, inspirational literature, walking, or calling a friend are options that readily come to mind. Anna also experiences guilt when she does nice things for herself so another assignment is buying herself flowers once a week. "Yes, I can do that. That feels right." For Anna, these assignments won't be easy, but they will feel right and they will build upon themselves slowly, over time becoming more ingrained.

All change processes, whether we are talking about addiction, healing a relationship, or personal growth, involve interplay between forward steps and backward steps. In my work as a therapist, I continually have to remind discouraged clients that periodic regression to their default setting is an inevitable part of the process. It does not mean that their efforts are futile. I have to remind myself of this as well. It is very easy to lose heart along the way and give ourselves up for lost. The grip that homeostasis exerts is part of what gives our world and our bodies their predictability and comfort. And this is also what makes attempts to change so terribly frustrating. Forgetting is natural. It is a product of the invisible hold that "our way of doing things" has over us. We forget what is possible, and we forget what inspires us to remember this.

What does this mean, then, regarding your efforts to change, to become healthier and more mindful around food? It means this: as you go along your change process, prepare to also go backward. The key to successful change is measured by your ability to re-mind yourself of your goals and recommit to using your tools over and over and over again. Remember the words "resolve" and "refrain" used in Pema Chödrön's impulse control formula. Over and over and over again. What you will notice as you continue this dialectic of remembering and forgetting is that the gap between forgetting and remembering will get smaller and smaller. So, where it might have taken you three months to remember that you feel better when you eat more healthfully, it may take three weeks, then three days, then three hours, three minutes, three seconds, "Oh, yes, I remember how good that feels." It is the small, seemingly incidental things that accumulate over time that you can use to keep yourself conscious and aware throughout your day. Setting aside a time for meditation, journaling, connecting with nature, or reaching out to a friend are all examples of activities that you can use to reorient yourself at any time. As these patterns build momentum in your life, they become habits rather than chores.

Reflections to Re-Mind Yourself

1. What tools help you to remember your higher intentions for yourself? Books, inspirational speakers, and certain friends can work as reminders.

2. How can you integrate more re-minders into your daily life that will keep you conscious of the vital role food plays in creating more health and vitality in your life?

In-Sight—Working with Deep Habits (Samskaras)

In-sight literally means turning your gaze inward. It is a practice of developing intimacy with your interior world. The capacity to Witness, or study, your own behavior is called svadhaya in yogic terminology, which means "self study." It requires the mild dislocation of perspective that we have been discussing throughout this chapter. Instead of being captured by your experience, you step a bit to the side so that you can see yourself in action. Through this more objective perspective, you begin to notice the patterns of behavior and beliefs that rule your consciousness. Developing the ability to watch yourself is one of the primary functions of therapy, and it can also be cultivated through yoga and meditation. When you become a better observer of yourself, you can initiate change because you are more objective about your behavior, rather than clinging fiercely to your old habits simply because it is your way of doing things. You make choices that cut through the fabric of your conditioning. The "momentary pause between cause and effect" becomes hard-wired into your consciousness. In order to cultivate this pause, you must create space between yourself and your conditioned responses. This space between cause and effect is the space where the Witness resides. When you create more space in your consciousness, rather than filling it up with reactive thoughts and behaviors (which may include donuts!), you are able to obtain a clearer view of yourself and deepen your understanding of how you came to be who you are. This open space allows you to make more conscious choices about who you shall become, since you are not just blindly reenacting the past.

Developing insight is the process of looking into your mind and studying your patterns of behavior and how this reflects your particular conditioning. When you have only a vague sense of how your history has shaped you, you will be unprepared for the force of the ingrained habits and impulses that lay in your body-mind. When you have some awareness of your vulnerabilities and quirks and you can meet and greet yourself with some acceptance, you are far more able to interrupt your reactive habits and past conditioning. Then you are ready to tango with life on life's terms, rather than reenacting the memories of your past wounds in your current life. As you develop more objective interest in yourself, shame subsides. You are no longer defending your way of doing things or criticizing yourself for it. Rather, you are exploring your patterns and asking (to borrow a line from Dr. Phil), "How is this working for me?" If you decide that it is not working, then you can make a choice to change your behavior. This is not as easy as it sounds, as most of us know. In fact, as you study your conditioning, you may find that your habitual patterns/samskaras reach far deeper than your individual history. You may be living out a legacy that has ancestral roots, extending from you, to your parents, and beyond. Developing this level of insight into your conditioning widens your lens from yourself to include others from your history. Recognizing the legacy that you are acting out deepens your compassion, not only for yourself your own particular brand of suffering, but for the suffering of those who have preceded you.

Samantha is a tallish, slender woman in her mid-forties. Very driven in her life, she wears her fatigue in an intense gaze that is shrouded by deep circles around her eyes. Samantha came to therapy due to chronic anxiety about her health. She had recently had a collapse in her energy levels that forced her to pull back from her rigorous exercise program. This was a lifestyle shift that she found deeply disturbing. Samantha was very focused on her health and on maintaining a slender physique. Having suffered from bulimia in the past, she was terrified of being out of control around food and struggled fiercely to exert what control she could over her current body. The fact that she did not feel well, and did not know why, robbed her of this control. Samantha would spend hours ruminating over possible reasons for her fatigue and surf the internet in search of answers. She was highly attentive to any unfamiliar sensations in her body and would immediately conclude that she had cancer if she experienced any new lump, bump, or pain. These symptoms gave Samantha great anxiety and compromised her functioning as a wife and mother, let alone her ability to feel joy in her life.

Samantha's unhappiness was strong enough to open her up to the process of therapy. Although not naturally drawn to meditation, she was willing to try it when I explained how it could help her. She took it on in the way she took on other things in her life, with vigilance and determination, though not a lot of joy. Alongside her meditation practice, we explored her early life and the forces that shaped her as a child. Samantha's mother was a highly anxious, narcissistic woman. She was a loving mother at times, especially when Samantha was a young girl. Samantha shared warm memories of being cared for by her mother when she was ill and described her early childhood as a time of great safely and security derived from her mother's love. In spite of this security, Samantha was a fearful, anxious child. She had trouble going to school and would often be plagued with worry that her mother would die and leave her. In addition, when she was nine Samantha developed a significant phobia of vomiting. This fear would come up to sabotage her excitement whenever she was going to spend time away from her mother. At age fourteen, Samantha's vomiting phobia transmuted into bulimia. She never purged due to her fear of vomiting, but she would eat compulsively and then diet and exercise to undo the evidence. This pattern continued for six years until she received treatment in her early twenties from a gifted therapist. "She saved my life," she commented with great feeling when discussing the role this therapist had in her development.

As Samantha's anxiety lessened and her meditation practice deepened, she developed more insight into her pattern of fear and anxiety around her body. "I realize that I have not felt safe in my body since I was nine years old. I have always felt as though something was wrong inside." Samantha realized that her fears about her health were not about this or that ache or pain, but rather reflected her deeper fear that her body was somehow damaged or unsafe. "My worst fear is that something is wrong with me and somehow I did it to myself." She added that this fear was coupled with anticipation of being excoriated by her mother for her self-neglect or carelessness. Somehow her condition would be deemed her own fault and she would be left alone to suffer. Her exploration of her anxiety opened the door for her to examine the deeper samskaras at play in her issues. Samantha's mother had lost her own mother to ovarian cancer when she was twelve years old. She was left to be raised by a cruel, and at times sadistic, father who seemingly took pleasure in humiliating his sensitive and grief-stricken daughter. Samantha realized that her distrust of her body was an invisible legacy derived from her mother's early abandonment by her own mother. The fear of something wrong inside was something Samantha's mother also struggled with. Though she shared little with her daughter about her fears, Samantha knew her mother was terrified of getting cancer as well. Samantha began to feel more compassion for her mother, and for herself, as her understanding deepened about the role that loss and illness played in their shared ancestry. This gave Samantha a wider perspective on her own symptoms. She realized that in some ways she was creating what she most feared—by driving her body to perform through exercise, she was creating illness and making her worst fears come true. Bulimia was the perfect metaphor for her control issues of doing and undoing. She would create distress by bingeing and then get rid of the distress by exercising and not eating. In this way, she acted out her control issues—after all, she was creating her own distress and then fixing it. This was her solution to the human dilemma of living in a vulnerable body that can and will get sick. Her "solution" was also creating the very thing she dreaded—it was making her sick. The clarity of perspective that Samantha gained from her meditation and therapy allowed her to relax into the present state of her body and to respond more sensitively to her body's needs. Eventually she regained some energy and was able to resume a more moderate exercise program that was respectful of her actual capacity, rather than a prescribed amount that was predetermined by her Egoic-self/ahamkara.

Reflections on Your Conditioning

1. Reflect for a few minutes on your particular conditioning about food and your body. What messages did your parents either implicitly or explicitly convey?

2. Now reflect on your parents' conditioning. What milieu were they steeped in as they developed? Does this increase your compassion for them?

Patience with the Process

Many of my female clients have shared with me the integral role their body plays in their well-being. Feeling "fat," or gaining weight, can sabotage their mood regardless of what is going well in the rest of their life. The flip side of this fixation is complete repression of the body, wherein the body exists alongside the mind but there is little conscious awareness given to the physical being. Either side of this polarity is no way to live—we are, after all, embodied creatures. Often individuals swing between the two polarities—either fixating on the physical state of the body with the intent to "fix" (dieting for example), or conversely, repressing the feeling body in search of ways to numb—enter extreme eating or alcohol use. In both cases, the mind lands on the concrete domain of the body and seeks either to change the outside through intervention or manage the inside by numbing. Both sides of the polarity are a byproduct of dissociation from one's present living body.

Given the significant challenges of being human (we are all going to die, are we not?), is it any wonder that we bear down on and seek a remedy to our problems on the material plane of the body? It is easy to be fixated on the concrete with simplistic notions that if we fix or change something in the domain of the physical body/annamayakosa, we will be relieved and renewed. Our Egoic-self easily perpetuates this fantasy. And when you are controlled by your Egoic-self, you become enslaved by commands to fix and change your body, your home, and your hair. And doesn't our culture reinforce this fixation with every commercial and enticement that is hurled our way on a daily basis? You must use your intelligence, buddhi, in order to not be yo-yo'd about by the simplistic whims to achieve this or that change on the surface level. The process involves slow changes over time and slow reintegration of your aware-ness (your mind—your Clever-mind, Egoic-self, and Witness working with your physical being).

Individuals with food disorders have hooked into food (or lack thereof, in the case of restrictors) as a solution to discomfort. This is not a conscious decision—it's a pattern that has taken root in the body-mind in response to pain that had no relational solution. Emotional pain in childhood when the child feels isolated, abandoned, or shamed by key people and has no alternative but to go to for soothing, sets the stage for a reliance on a sub-stance to cover over feelings of abandonment. Emotional abandonment is a wretched, psychologically disorienting, even terrifying experience. Addic-tion takes root here, in this moment of great need, or repeated moments of great need, that go unmet (unsated, so to speak). The young child "decides" (not consciously, of course) that the world of human others is dangerous, unpredictable, and painful. In order to have some means of comfort, some-thing else must take the place of secure relationship with others. Enter food (or any addiction). The pleasure and soothing associated with food becomes magnified and distorted since it is taking the place of something far more primal, the need for comforting and soothing from others. Food addic-tion is caused by the ongoing repetition of using food to soothe, to create meaning, and to facilitate anchoring. There is a strong psycho-physiological hook, a samskara (think deep grooves) that lives in your body-mind. This habitual pattern/samskara is workable. You can create new grooves. The first step is making your current habit/samskara very conscious. You are encouraged to feel it fully—feel your desire to eat, get interested in the edges of your hunger, your use of food to mark time and buffer experience. And then you become willing to experiment with the boundaries of your need.

This book has given you some ideas and suggestions to begin this process and to explore how yoga and meditation can provide a path for you to follow. The yoga of food is based on the idea that we start with simple changes grounded in the material world and that the process will take on its own momentum over time. It will feel overwhelming at first and so it is important to pace yourself and start with small changes that you can build upon. Remember resistance, remember regression. These are all normal aspects of our shared human experience and our tendency to cling to what we know. If you are aware of your inevitable resistance and the inevitability of regression, they need not be saboteurs of progress, but instead known entities along the way that you can cope with sensibly and without turning against yourself and giving up.

Recommended Resources

Yoga

Baptiste, Baron. *40 Days to Personal Revolution. A Breakthrough Program to Radically Change Your Body and Awaken the Sacred Within Your Soul.* New York: Fireside Books, 2004.

————*The Yoga Bootcamp Box: An Interactive Program to Revolutionize Your Life with Yoga.* New York: St. Martin's Griffin, 2004. Audio CD.

Corn, Seane. *Vinyasa Flow Yoga: Uniting Movement and Breath.* Boulder, CO: Gaiam, Inc. DVD.

Farhi, Donna. *The Breathing Book: Good Health and Vitality Through Essential Breath Work.* New York: Holt Paperbacks, 1996.

Iyengar, B.K.S. *Light on Life: The Yoga Journey to Wholeness, Inner Peace and Ultimate Freedom.* New York: Rodale Books, 2005.

————*Light on Yoga: Yoga Dipika.* New York: Schocken Books, 1966.

Kaminoff, Leslie. *Breath Centered Yoga.* 2010. Compact Disc.

Lasater, Judith. *Relax and Renew: Restful Yoga for Stressful Times.* Berkeley, CA: Rodnell Press, 1995.

Lentz, Abby. *HeavyWeight Yoga 2: Change the Image of Yoga.* Austin, TX: Heartfelt Yoga LLC. Audio CD.

Meditation/Mindfulness

Chödrön, Pema. *Getting Unstuck. Breaking Your Habitual Patterns & Encountering Naked Reality.* Boulder, CO: Sounds True, Inc., 2005.

———*Good Medicine: How to Turn Pain into Compassion with Tonglen Meditation.* Boulder, CO: Sounds True, Inc., 2001.

———*Pure Meditation: The Tibetan Buddhist Practice of Inner Peace.* Boulder, CO: Sounds True Inc., 2000.

Salzberg, Sharon. *Real Happiness: The Power of Meditation.* New York: Workman Publishing Co. Inc., 2011.

Weil, Andrew. *Breathing: The Master Key to Self-Healing.* Boulder, CO: Sounds True Inc., 1999.

Nutrition/Food

Kessler, David, *The End of Overeating: Taking Control of the Insatiable American Appetite.* New York: Rodale Books, 2009.

Pollan, Michael. *In Defense of Food: An Eater's Manifesto.* New York: Penguin Group, 2008.

Integrative Approaches to Food and Body Image

Bays, Jan Chozen. *Mindful Eating: A Guide to Rediscovering a Healthy and Joyful Relationship with Food.* Boston, MA: Shambhala, 2009.

Roth, Geneen. *Feeding the Hungry Heart: The Experience of Compulsive Eating.* Indianapolis, IN: Bobbs-Merrill, 1982.

———*Women Food and God: An Unexpected Path to Almost Everything.* New York: Scribner, 2010.

Seller, Christine. *Yoga from the Inside Out: Making Peace with Your Body Through Yoga.* Prescott, AZ: Hohm Press, 2003.

Integrative Psychology

Cope, Stephen. *Yoga and the Quest for the True Self.* New York: Bantam Books, 1999.

Forbes, Bo. *Yoga for Emotional Balance: Simple Practices to Help Relieve Anxiety and Depression.* Boston, MA: Shambhala Publications, 2011.

Harris, Russ. *The Happiness Trap: How to Stop Struggling and Start Living.* Boston, MA: Shambhala Publications, 2007.

Judith, Anodea. *Eastern Body, Western Mind: Psychology and the Chakra System as a Path to the Self.* Berkeley, CA: Celestial Arts, 2004.

Siegel, Daniel. *Mindsight: The New Science of Personal Transformation.* New York: Bantam Books, 2010.

Glossary

Ahamkara: The Egoic-self, or "I-maker." We identify this as who we are, yet this is misguided because it leads to a feeling of separation. The yogic path inspires a sense of non-separation from all that exists.

Ahimsa: A yogic principle referring to the value of non-violence in both thought and behavior.

Anandamaya kosa: The fifth layer of your Being, your "Bliss body." This is the level of universal consciousness, of non-separation with all that is. Reaching this level of awareness is the ultimate goal of yoga.

Annamaya kosa: Your physical body, inside and out. According to yoga philosophy, it is the first layer of your Being, which consists of five layered bodies moving from gross (material) to subtle.

Buddhi: The part of you that learns to act on your own behalf and that has the capacity for insight and self-reflection.

Chitta: The part of your mind related to memory and will. Chitta allows you to make decisions.

Karma: In Classical Yoga philosophy, karma refers to the hold that past actions, even from past lives, have on us. It is undesirable and the goal of yoga is to free ourselves by nullifying desire. In this book, the term is used in a more casual way to refer to the power of cause and effect.

Kleshas: Obstacles to clear seeing. These refer to the five common pitfalls that lead to unclear seeing and unskillful living. Unclear seeing, attraction, aversion, ego, and fear are the five kleshas.

Manomaya kosa: The third layer of your Being, referring to your everyday mind. This is the "clever" part of you that problem solves and is oriented toward short-term gratifications.

Mitri: A practice from Buddhist psychology that cultivates loving kindness toward the self and all Beings.

Namaste: A salutation meaning "the light in me sees the light in you." Traditionally said at the end of a yoga class.

Pranamaya kosa: The second layer of your Being, referring to your energetic body. The branch of yoga devoted to breath (pranayama) works with this level of your body. According to yogic philosophy, your energetic body is every bit as real as your physical body.

Samskaras: A yogic term referring to the power that our habitual patterns have in creating and maintaining our material, energetic, and spiritual qualities.

Savasana: Also known as corpse pose, this is the final rest at the end of a yoga class where you let go of all effort and absorb the benefits of your practice.

Tapas: A yogic practice of applying heat, or gentle discipline, to ourselves in order to create positive change.

Ujaiyi breath: A form of yogic breathing that helps cultivate regulation of the breath. It is nasal breathing coupled with a mild constriction in the throat that creates a subtle oceanic sound.

Vijnanamaya kosa: The fourth layer of your Being, referring to your Wisdom body. This is the part of you that is connected to universal intelligence and can help free you from identification with your ego.

Witness: The aspect of your consciousness that is able to observe yourself with some objectivity. In Western psychology this is called the observing ego.

Bibliography

Chödrön, Pema. *Getting Unstuck. Breaking Your Habitual Patterns &* *Encountering Naked Reality.* Boulder, CO: Sounds True Inc., 2005.

Delaney, Lisa, *The Secrets of a Former Fat Girl: How to Lose Two, Four (or More!) Dress Sizes and Find Yourself Along the Way.* New York: Penguin Group, 2007.

Horton, Carol. *Yoga Ph.D.: Integrating the Life of the Mind and the Wisdom of the Body.* Chicago: Kleio Books, 2012.

Iyengar, B.K.S. *Light on Life: The Yoga Journey to Wholeness, Inner Peace and Ultimate Freedom.* New York: Rodale Books, 2005.

Kessler, David, *The End of Overeating: Taking Control of the Insatiable American Appetite.* New York: Rodale Books, 2009.

Kornfield, Jack, and Daniel Siegel. *Mindfulness and the Brain: A Professional Training in the Science & Practice of Meditative Awareness.* Boulder, CO: Sounds True, Inc., 2010.

Kuffel, Frances. *Passing for Thin: Losing Half My Weight and Finding Myself.* New York: Broadway Books, 2004.

Pollan, Michael. *In Defense of Food: An Eater's Manifesto.* New York: Penguin Books, 2008.

Siegel, Daniel. *Mindsight: The New Science of Personal Transformation.* New York: Bantam Books, 2010.

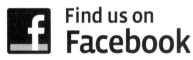
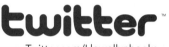

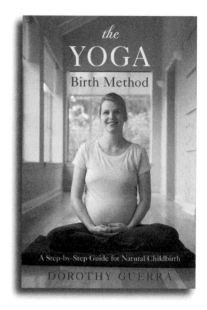

The Yoga Birth Method
A Step-by-Step Guide for Natural Childbirth
DOROTHY GUERRA

Plan a childbirth that's calm, natural, and enlightened. *The Yoga Birth Method* is an empowering eight-step pathway to achieving a positive and joyful birth experience.

Applying the wisdom of yoga to childbirth, Dorothy Guerra offers a solid plan for managing the mind, body, and spirit throughout the stages of pregnancy and labor. Couples choose an intention that becomes a focal point for embracing a calm state of mind throughout the physical and emotional challenges of childbirth. You'll discover what to expect during each stage of labor and how to manage pain, eliminate anxiety, and encourage labor progression with breathing techniques and yoga poses. There's also guidance in drafting a birth plan, labor-support techniques for birth partners, information on medical intervention, and a "go to" chapter with checklists to use when the big day arrives.

978-0-7387-3665-5, 240 pp., 6 x 9   **$15.99**

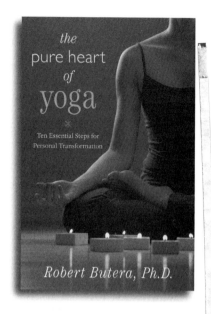

the
pure heart
of
yoga

Ten Essential Steps for
Personal Transformation

Robert Butera, Ph.D.

The Pure Heart of Yoga
Ten Essential Steps for Personal Transformation
ROBERT BUTERA, PHD

Connect to the infinite through yoga and experience true transformation on the physical, emotional, psychological, and spiritual planes.

This inspiring book teaches yoga the way the original masters envisioned it—a holistic union of body, mind, and spirit. Dr. Butera's simple ten-step approach invites all levels of yoga practitioners and teachers to deepen their understanding of yoga philosophy and work toward health and self-realization. By cultivating a mindful practice of the yoga postures, you will learn to balance emotions, focus the mind, control breathing, work with the body's energy centers (chakras), eliminate psychological blocks, and create a sense of purpose and peace for life.

978-0-7387-1487-5, 336 pp., 6 x 9   **$21.95**

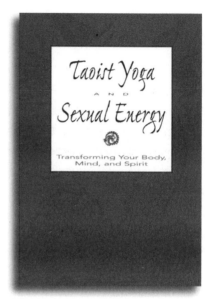

Taoist Yoga and Sexual Energy
Eric Steven Yudelove

When most people think of the term yoga, they think of the body-stretching techniques from India. But there are many different forms of yoga, including techniques practiced in secret by the Taoist masters in the Far East. Some of the most important, yet previously secret techniques of Taoist Alchemy and Sexual Kung Fu are revealed for the first time by Taoist Master Eric Steven Yudelove in *Taoist Yoga and Sexual Energy*.

This is not just a book, it is an entire, fourteen-week course in alchemy, healing, and magick. Perhaps the most important part of this is learning how to manipulate the body's mysterious energies. In order to do this you will learn many breathing techniques, including hair breathing, reverse breathing, bone marrow breathing, and several more. You'll learn the amazing secrets of Chi Gung, including standing, sitting, lying, and moving forms.

As the title of the book shows, this book is also about working with the sexual energy. You will learn breathing techniques, visualizations, and massage methods that will allow you and your partner to experience bliss beyond your wildest imagination!

978-1-56718-834-9, 312 pp., 7 x 10   **$27.95**

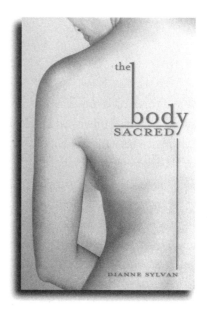

The Body Sacred
DIANNE SYLVAN

When you look in the mirror, do you see a Goddess? For anyone who's experienced a "fat day" or wished a doctor could make them younger, Wiccan Dianne Sylvan speaks candidly about overcoming body hatred and offers a spiritual path back to Divine femininity.

Sharing her own struggles with poor body image and self-acceptance, Sylvan explores how the impossible standard of female beauty has developed and endured. Emphasizing the Mother, the Healer, the Lover, and other archetypes of one's relationship with the sacred body, the author provides a uniquely Wiccan approach to achieving a healthy, new self-perception as Goddess.

978-0-7387-0761-7, 312 pp., 6 x 9   **$22.99**

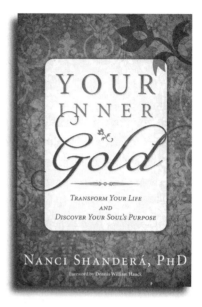

Your Inner Gold
Transform Your Life and Discover Your Soul's Purpose
Nanci Shanderá, PhD

Create positive personal life changes, free yourself from fear, and open your heart to the shining Philosopher's Stone of *Your Inner Gold*. This alchemical guide presents a comprehensive model to help you discover your true self and its relationship to your soul's purpose.

Transform yourself with the seven basic stages of spiritual alchemy: calcination, dissolution, separation, conjunction, putrefaction-fermentation, mortification, distillation, and coagulation. Whether you're new to spiritual practice or an advanced seeker, this useful guide will help you apply each principle to your life through meditations, exercises, and other creative techniques. Learn how to overcome what holds you back, how your soul speaks to you, how your soul's pre-birth agreements affect your life challenges, and much more. Even though you can't remove any aspect of yourself, you can transform it with spiritual alchemy.

978-0-7387-3601-3, 240 pp., 6 x 9   **$15.99**